METHODS IN MOLECULAR BIOLOGY

Series Editor
John M. Walker
School of Life and Medical Sciences
University of Hertfordshire
Hatfield, Hertfordshire, UK

For further volumes:
http://www.springer.com/series/7651

For over 35 years, biological scientists have come to rely on the research protocols and methodologies in the critically acclaimed *Methods in Molecular Biology* series. The series was the first to introduce the step-by-step protocols approach that has become the standard in all biomedical protocol publishing. Each protocol is provided in readily-reproducible step-by step fashion, opening with an introductory overview, a list of the materials and reagents needed to complete the experiment, and followed by a detailed procedure that is supported with a helpful notes section offering tips and tricks of the trade as well as troubleshooting advice. These hallmark features were introduced by series editor Dr. John Walker and constitute the key ingredient in each and every volume of the *Methods in Molecular Biology* series. Tested and trusted, comprehensive and reliable, all protocols from the series are indexed in PubMed.

The Olfactory System

Edited by

Bradley J. Goldstein

Department of Head and Neck Surgery & Communication Sciences, Duke University School of Medicine, Durham, NC, USA; Department of Neurobiology, Duke University School of Medicine, Durham, NC, USA

Hiroaki Matsunami

Department of Molecular Genetics and Microbiology, Duke University School of Medicine, Durham, NC, USA; Department of Neurobiology, Duke University School of Medicine, Durham, NC, USA

Humana Press

Editors
Bradley J. Goldstein
Department of Head and Neck Surgery
& Communication Sciences
Duke University School of Medicine
Durham, NC, USA

Department of Neurobiology
Duke University School of Medicine
Durham, NC, USA

Hiroaki Matsunami
Department of Molecular Genetics and Microbiology
Duke University School of Medicine
Durham, NC, USA

Department of Neurobiology
Duke University School of Medicine
Durham, NC, USA

ISSN 1064-3745 ISSN 1940-6029 (electronic)
Methods in Molecular Biology
ISBN 978-1-0716-3427-1 ISBN 978-1-0716-3425-7 (eBook)
https://doi.org/10.1007/978-1-0716-3425-7

Cover Caption: Mouse olfactory neurons, labeled with fluorescent reporter (yellow), from lab of Brad Goldstein.

This Humana imprint is published by the registered company Springer Science+Business Media, LLC, part of Springer Nature.
The registered company address is: 1 New York Plaza, New York, NY 10004, U.S.A.

Paper in this product is recyclable.

Preface

The mammalian olfactory system detects and discriminates volatile odor molecules that are essential for various activities, including identification of food, avoidance of predators or environmental hazards, and identification of mating partners. In humans, olfaction also contributes to the hedonic qualities of food and beverage intake, and impaired olfactory function can have severe consequences, including depression, malnutrition, and increased mortality in the elderly. Olfactory dysfunction can result from various clinical conditions, and the COVID-19 pandemic has been strongly associated with anosmia and parosmia, with incomplete recovery noted in some cases. However, there are currently no effective treatments for disorders that damage the olfactory system, emphasizing the need for ongoing research to understand the physiology and pathophysiology of olfaction.

The olfactory system comprises both peripheral and central structures. The olfactory mucosa in the nasal cavity houses the somata of the primary olfactory sensory neurons, as well as key supporting populations, including sustentacular and microvillar cells, basal stem cells, and Bowman's glands. Olfactory sensory neurons are activated when odor molecules interact with olfactory receptors at their cilia membrane, and they project axons via Cranial Nerve I to synapse at the glomerular layer of the olfactory bulbs. Central processing and coding of olfactory perceptions occur via projection to additional areas, including the piriform cortex and amygdala. This volume's contributors have expertise in investigating key aspects of biology in the olfactory system from the periphery to the cortex.

Several chapters in this volume address experimental techniques for studying cell populations in the olfactory mucosa. Chapter 1 describes techniques for manipulating and measuring olfactory cilia function. Chapter 2 discusses an approach for investigating spatial RNA expression in olfactory mucosa. Chapter 3 provides approaches for optical activation and measurement of TRP channels, an area of active study in the olfactory periphery. Chapter 4 describes an approach for precise monitoring of mouse respiration. The olfactory mucosa is not only a chemosensory organ but also a key barrier structure; therefore, immune cell populations and their interactions with olfactory cells are of importance. Chapter 5 discusses the identification of immune populations in olfactory tissue.

Mechanistic insights into olfactory sensory neuron function require the use and refinement of advanced techniques. In Chapter 6, the use of chromatin immunoprecipitation with olfactory neurons is discussed in detail. Chapter 7 provides a discussion of an in vivo approach to label and identify activated olfactory neurons combining phospho-S6 immunohistochemistry and fluorescent RNA in situ hybridization. Many approaches have been applied to understanding specific odorant-olfactory receptor interactions. Chapter 8 discusses approaches to measure the cell surface expression of olfactory receptors in heterologous cell systems. Chapter 9 reviews an approach for the FACS purification of mouse olfactory neurons. Efforts to translate discoveries to clinical application require the use of human samples. Chapter 10 discusses approaches for obtaining and processing olfactory mucosal biopsies from human patients.

Several chapters focus attention on the olfactory bulbs and cortex. Chapter 11 discusses the use of optical recording in the mouse olfactory bulb for acute or chronic experiments, which can be coupled with viral delivery of specific fluorescent sensors. Several methods for exploring spatial transcriptomics have been developed recently. Chapter 12 provides an approach for mapping olfactory receptor expression in olfactory bulb using target capture of mRNA preparations, and Chapter 13 discusses an approach for visualization of gene expression in the mouse olfactory bulb, termed Slide-SeqV2. Mouse genetic approaches involving inducible Cre-loxP systems are powerful techniques that permit visualization and manipulation of gene expression in a cell type-specific manner. Chapter 14 discusses the inducible labeling of mitral cells with tamoxifen administration. General approaches for olfactory tissue staining are reviewed in Chapter 15. Finally, Chapter 16 provides an overview of approaches for multi-region recording in the mouse olfactory system using opto-tagging combined with multielectrode arrays.

Together, this volume covers a wide array of approaches currently useful for investigating molecular biology and physiology in the peripheral and central olfactory system. The application of these approaches to address key unanswered questions will be helpful in understanding both normal function and pathobiology, ultimately providing novel treatment approaches for human olfactory disorders.

Durham, NC, USA

Bradley J. Goldstein
Hiroaki Matsunami

Contents

Contributors

JANARDHAN P. BHATTARAI • *Department of Neuroscience, University of Pennsylvania Perelman School of Medicine, Philadelphia, PA, USA*

KEVIN A. BOLDING • *Department of Neurobiology, Duke University, Durham, NC, USA; Monell Chemical Senses Center, Philadelphia, PA, USA; Department of Neuroscience, University of Pennsylvania, Philadelphia, PA, USA*

MARCO BRONDI • *Veneto Institute of Molecular Medicine, Fondazione per la Ricerca Biomedica Avanzata, Padova, Italy; IN-CNR, Padova, Italy*

RHEA CHOI • *Department of Head and Neck Surgery & Communication Sciences, Duke University School of Medicine, Durham, NC, USA*

AI FANG • *Stowers Institute for Medical Research, Kansas City, MO, USA*

JOHN B. FINLAY • *Medical Scientist Training Program, Duke University School of Medicine, Durham, NC, USA*

KEVIN M. FRANKS • *Department of Neurobiology, Duke University, Durham, NC, USA*

XIAOCHEN FU • *Sensory and Behavioural Neuroscience Unit, Okinawa Institute of Science and Technology Graduate University, Okinawa, Japan*

IZUMI FUKUNAGA • *Sensory and Behavioural Neuroscience Unit, Okinawa Institute of Science and Technology Graduate University, Okinawa, Japan*

BRADLEY J. GOLDSTEIN • *Department of Head and Neck Surgery & Communication Sciences, Duke University School of Medicine, Durham, NC, USA; Department of Neurobiology, Duke University School of Medicine, Durham, NC, USA*

JULIEN C. HABIF • *Department of Pharmacology and Therapeutics, University of Florida College of Medicine, Gainesville, FL, USA; Center for Smell and Taste, University of Florida College of Medicine, Gainesville, FL, USA*

RALPH ABI HACHEM • *Department of Head and Neck Surgery & Communication Sciences, Duke University School of Medicine, Durham, NC, USA*

ERIC H. HOLBROOK • *Department of Otolaryngology—Head and Neck Surgery, Massachusetts Eye and Ear, Harvard Medical School, Boston, MA, USA*

YU-PEI HUANG • *Sensory and Behavioural Neuroscience Unit, Okinawa Institute of Science and Technology Graduate University, Okinawa, Japan*

DAVID JANG • *Department of Head and Neck Surgery & Communication Sciences, Duke University School of Medicine, Durham, NC, USA*

EMMA JANKE • *Department of Neuroscience, University of Pennsylvania Perelman School of Medicine, Philadelphia, PA, USA*

JEROME K. KAHIAPO • *Department of Molecular Biology and Biochemistry, Nelson Biological Laboratories, Rutgers, The State University of New Jersey, Piscataway, NJ, USA*

TIFFANY KO • *Department of Neurobiology, Duke University School of Medicine, Durham, NC, USA*

TRESE LEINDERS-ZUFALL • *Center for Integrative Physiology and Molecular Medicine (CIPMM), Saarland University, Homburg, Germany*

HUA LI • *Stowers Institute for Medical Research, Kansas City, MO, USA*

SANDER LINDEMAN • *Sensory and Behavioural Neuroscience Unit, Okinawa Institute of Science and Technology Graduate University, Okinawa, Japan*

CLAUDIA LODOVICHI • *Veneto Institute of Molecular Medicine, Fondazione per la Ricerca Biomedica Avanzata, Padova, Italy; IN-CNR, Padova, Italy; Padova Neuroscience Center, Padova, Italy*
MINGHONG MA • *Department of Neuroscience, University of Pennsylvania Perelman School of Medicine, Philadelphia, PA, USA*
LUCINDA MADDERA • *Stowers Institute for Medical Research, Kansas City, MO, USA*
ADAM MAGO • *Sensory and Behavioural Neuroscience Unit, Okinawa Institute of Science and Technology Graduate University, Okinawa, Japan*
MELANIE MAKHLOUF • *Sidra Medicine, Doha, Qatar*
SETH MALLOY • *Stowers Institute for Medical Research, Kansas City, MO, USA*
JEFFREY R. MARTENS • *Department of Pharmacology and Therapeutics, University of Florida College of Medicine, Gainesville, FL, USA; Center for Smell and Taste, University of Florida College of Medicine, Gainesville, FL, USA*
LISA S. MATHEW • *Sidra Medicine, Doha, Qatar*
HIROAKI MATSUNAMI • *Department of Molecular Genetics and Microbiology, Duke University Medical Center, Duke University School of Medicine, Durham, NC, USA; Department of Neurobiology, Duke Institute for Brain Sciences, Durham, NC, USA*
TIMOTHY S. MCCLINTOCK • *Department of Physiology, University of Kentucky, Lexington, KY, USA*
SEAN MCKINNEY • *Stowers Institute for Medical Research, Kansas City, MO, USA*
KEVIN MONAHAN • *Department of Molecular Biology and Biochemistry, Nelson Biological Laboratories, Rutgers, The State University of New Jersey, Piscataway, NJ, USA*
E. ASHLEY MOSEMAN • *Department of Integrative Immunobiology, Duke University School of Medicine, Durham, NC, USA*
EMAN ABOU MOUSSA • *Sidra Medicine, Doha, Qatar*
MAIRA HARUME NAGAI • *Department of Molecular Genetics and Microbiology, Duke University Medical Center, Durham, NC, USA*
HIRONOBU NISHIJIMA • *Department of Otolaryngology—Head and Neck Surgery, The University of Tokyo, Tokyo, Japan*
NAVIN K. OJHA • *Center for Integrative Physiology and Molecular Medicine (CIPMM), Saarland University, Homburg, Germany*
ANOJA PERERA • *Stowers Institute for Medical Research, Kansas City, MO, USA*
KAITLYN PETENTLER • *Stowers Institute for Medical Research, Kansas City, MO, USA*
MICHAEL PETERSON • *Stowers Institute for Medical Research, Kansas City, MO, USA*
ANDREW PRICE • *Stowers Institute for Medical Research, Kansas City, MO, USA*
JONATHON RUSSELL • *Stowers Institute for Medical Research, Kansas City, MO, USA*
LUIS R. SARAIVA • *Sidra Medicine, Doha, Qatar; College of Health and Life Sciences, Hamad Bin Khalifa University, Doha, Qatar; Monell Chemical Senses Center, Philadelphia, PA, USA*
TOMOKO SENGOKU • *Department of Physiology, University of Kentucky, Lexington, KY, USA*
JENNIFER L. STRANGE • *Department of Microbiology, Immunology, and Molecular Genetics, University of Kentucky, Lexington, KY, USA*
JEEVAN TEWARI • *Department of Molecular Genetics and Microbiology, Duke University School of Medicine, Durham, NC, USA*
WILLIAM B. TITLOW • *Department of Physiology, University of Kentucky, Lexington, KY, USA*
MCKENZIE TREESE • *Stowers Institute for Medical Research, Kansas City, MO, USA*
QIANG WANG • *Department of Physiology, University of Kentucky, Lexington, KY, USA*

YONGFU WANG • *Stowers Institute for Medical Research, Kansas City, MO, USA*
SEBASTIAN A. WELLFORD • *Department of Integrative Immunobiology, Duke University School of Medicine, Durham, NC, USA*
CHAO XIE • *Department of Pharmacology and Therapeutics, University of Florida College of Medicine, Gainesville, FL, USA; Center for Smell and Taste, University of Florida College of Medicine, Gainesville, FL, USA*
C. RON YU • *Stowers Institute for Medical Research, Kansas City, MO, USA; Department of Cell Biology and Physiology, University of Kansas Medical Center, Kansas City, KS, USA*
KEVIN W. ZHU • *Department of Molecular Genetics and Microbiology, Duke University School of Medicine, Durham, NC, USA*
FRANK ZUFALL • *Center for Integrative Physiology and Molecular Medicine (CIPMM), Saarland University, Homburg, Germany*

Chapter 1

Visualizing and Manipulating Olfactory Cilia Through Viral Delivery Coupled with En Face Imaging of Intact OE

Julien C. Habif, Chao Xie, and Jeffrey R. Martens

Abstract

Olfactory cilia are the obligate transducers of the odorant signal, and thus their study has been a focus of investigation in the olfactory field. Various methodologies have been established to visualize the cilia of olfactory sensory neurons; however, these approaches are limited to static imaging and often lack the ability to resolve individual cilia projecting from solitary neurons in the postnatal mouse. Here we detail a procedure of the visualization of olfactory cilia by ectopic expression of fluorescently tagged proteins. The procedure can be used for the observation and manipulation of the olfactory cilia and ciliary proteins in both static and dynamic conditions.

Key words Cilia, Intranasal delivery, En face imaging, TIRF, FRAP, Olfactory epithelium

1 Introduction

In 1954, the first report of olfactory cilia was conducted using light and electron microscopy and demonstrated numerous, long cilia emanating from the dendritic endings of olfactory sensory neurons (OSNs) [1]. Early electron microscopy (EM) studies contributed to the vast majority of our current understanding of the morphology of olfactory cilia in various animal models, including rodents [2, 3], dogs [4, 5], reptiles [6, 7], and fish [8, 9]. Since then, technological advances have allowed dynamic processes in cilia to be measured such as protein transport [10–12] as well as the ability to ascertain mechanisms of dysfunction in ciliary diseases [10, 13–15]. The various methods employed to assess olfactory cilia possess advantages along with limitations that need to be considered when designing an experiment. Specifically, the type of microscopy (light or electron microscopy), the orientation of the tissue (coronal or en face), and the method for labeling (coating with

Authors "Julien C. Habif" and "Chao Xie" have equally contributed to this chapter.

Bradley J. Goldstein and Hiroaki Matsunami (eds.), *The Olfactory System*, Methods in Molecular Biology, vol. 2710,
https://doi.org/10.1007/978-1-0716-3425-7_1,

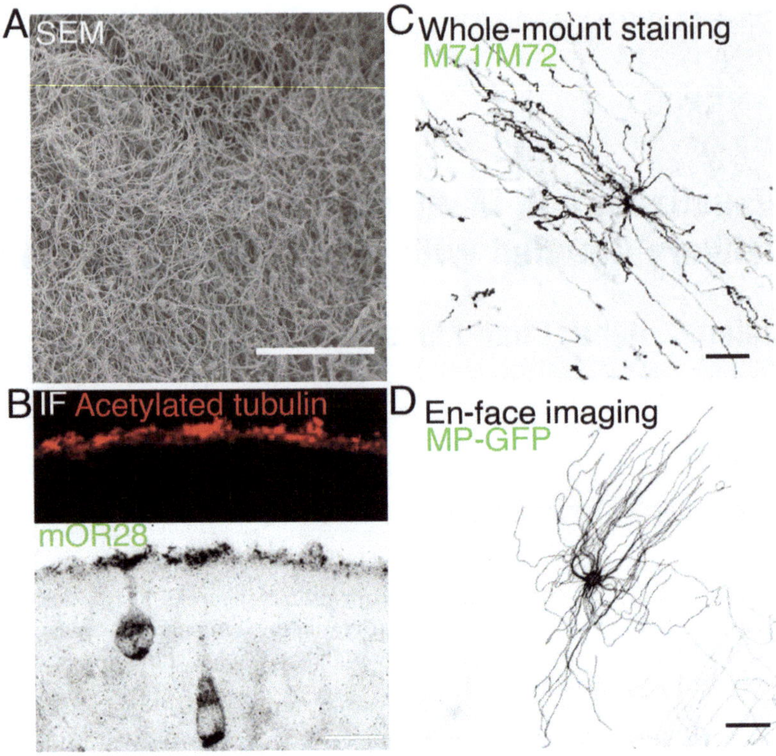

Fig. 1 Methods for visualizing the morphology of olfactory cilia. (**a**–**d**) Images of cilia from OSNs in mice utilizing different tissue orientations, labeling, and imaging techniques. (**a**) Representative scanning electron micrograph (SEM) of the surface of the OE. Scale 50 μm. (**b**) Representative immunofluorescent (IF) coronal section of the OE labeled for acetylated tubulin (top) and the odorant receptor, mOR28 (bottom). (**c**) Representative image of olfactory cilia using whole-mount staining. The OE was stained with an anti-M71/M72 antibody. (**d**) Representative live en face image of ectopically expressed AV-MP-GFP, demarking olfactory cilia of an individual OSN. Scale 10 μm

conductive material, immunolabeling, or virally delivering fluorescent probes) all need to be considered. For instance, transmission electron microscopy is most commonly used to examine the ultrastructure of cilia as it provides tremendous resolving power enabling the examination of the ciliary axoneme [2, 3]. Scanning electron microscopy (SEM) has been the predominant method for ciliary morphology analysis during embryogenesis (Fig. 1a). Fluorescence light microscopy of immunolabeled coronal sections of the nasal cavity is another method routinely used to assess ciliation and ciliary signaling protein distribution (Fig. 1b) [16]. Since both of these methods ubiquitously mark cilia, analysis of overall ciliation can be performed; however, in the postnatal animal olfactory, cilia form a dense meshwork making it impossible to distinguish cilia from individual OSNs. A method that circumvents this limitation is

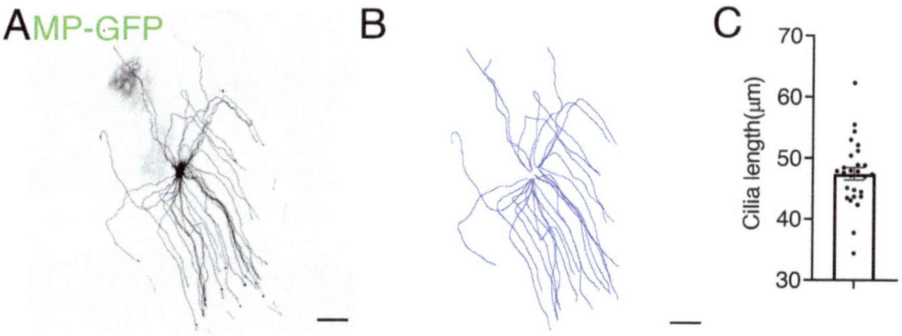

Fig. 2 Cilia length measurement using en face imaging. (**a**) Representative en face microscopy image of ectopically expressed MP-GFP in olfactory cilia under static conditions in a mouse. (**b**) Representative freehand line drawings of olfactory cilia. (**c**) Quantification of olfactory cilia length. Scale 10 μm

en face en bloc fluorescence imaging also referred to as whole-mount staining of the olfactory epithelium (OE) for a specific odorant receptor (OR) (Fig. 1c). However, whole-mount staining requires extreme care as tissue fixation can make the fragile olfactory cilia more vulnerable to physical damage during processing or imaging and limit assessment to a specific subpopulation of OSNs. These three methods outlined above to assess cilia morphology all require the fixation of tissue samples and therefore prevent the analysis of dynamic processes and additionally can cause artifacts due to sample processing.

This chapter describes a detailed methodology allowing the visualization and manipulation of olfactory cilia at a high resolution by coupling adenoviral transduction of fluorescent proteins and en face fluorescence imaging of the OE in live tissue [13]. The ability to control the infection rate through tittering the virus, and repeat delivery allows cilia from individual OSNs to be resolved and therefore permits the quantitative analysis of ciliation (Figs. 1d and 2a). The stochastic variation in infectivity results in the sampling of OSNs throughout the OE that does not discriminate based upon subpopulation of OSN. Beyond delineating olfactory cilia, this method allows dynamic ciliary processes to be measured, such as protein trafficking within a cilium by live-cell imaging with total internal reflection fluorescence (TIRF) microscopy (Fig. 3) [10, 12] and protein transport into the cilium with fluorescence recovery after photobleaching (FRAP) (Fig. 4) [17, 18]. Additionally, probes (i.e., GCaMP) or other proteins normally excluded from the cilium can be exogenously targeted to the cilia with a ciliary targeting motif [19]. Also, this technique allows for the manipulation of cilia by ectopic expression of proteins such as dominant negative proteins to assay the role of the protein [20],

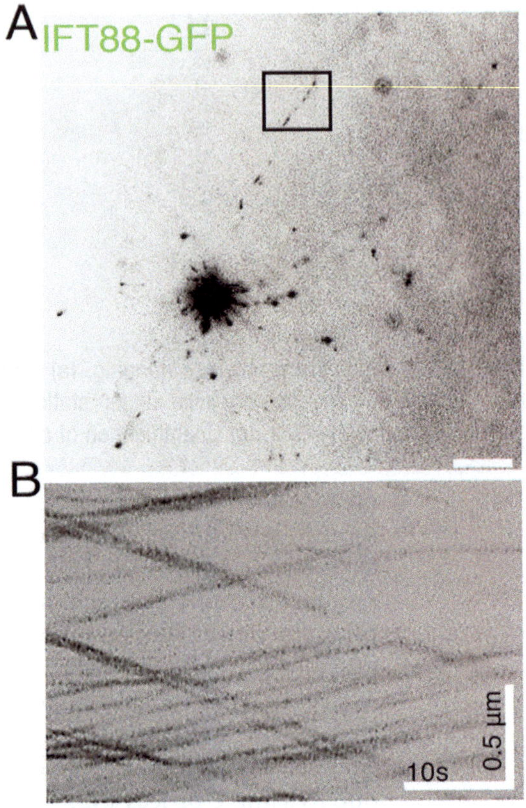

Fig. 3 Ciliary protein dynamics using Total Internal Reflection Fluorescence (TIRF) microscopy. (**a**) Representative en face TIRF microscopy image of ectopically expressed IFT88 tagged with a fluorescent protein (IFT88-GFP) in olfactory cilia in a mouse. Scale 10 μm. (**b**) Representative kymogram of IFT88-GFP trafficking in an OSN cilium. Scale 0.5 μm by 10 s

the photo-activatable adenylate cyclase bPAC to alter the activation of signal transduction cascades [21] or NP-EGTA to uncage Ca^{2+} [22]. En face fluorescence imaging alongside intranasal viral delivery has allowed for the elucidation of mechanisms of olfactory dysfunction induced by genetic mutations of ciliary proteins that cause a class of hereditary disorders, termed ciliopathies [10–12, 14, 15, 23, 24]. In summary, this technique allows for the (1) visualization of cilia from individual OSNs, (2) targeting probes to cilia, (3) manipulation of ciliary pathways, (4) assaying of dynamic ciliary processes, and (5) providing of mechanistic insight into ciliopathy-induced olfactory dysfunction. The following paper describes a detailed methodology of intranasally delivering virus to mice, tissue preparation of the olfactory turbinates, and imaging of olfactory cilia under static and dynamic (FRAP, TIRF) conditions.

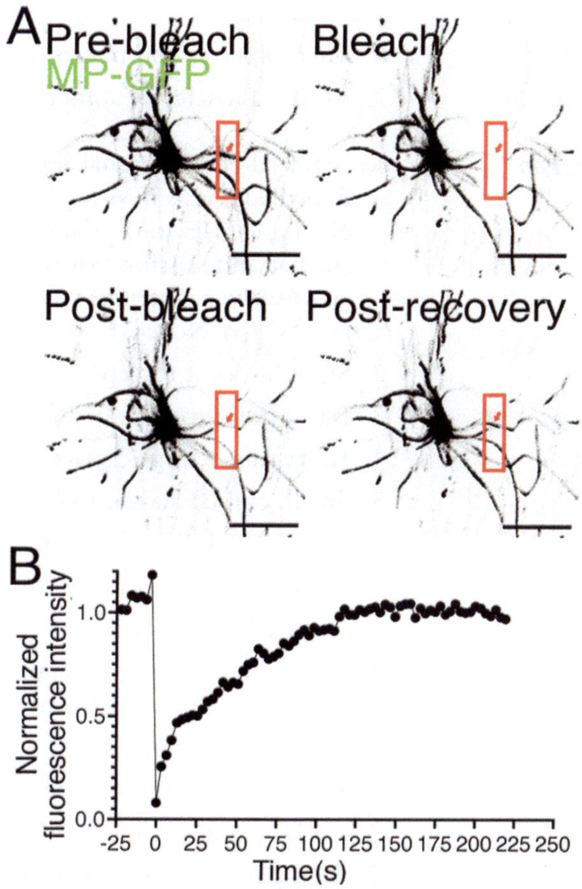

Fig. 4 Fluorescence recovery after photobleaching (FRAP) of olfactory cilia. (**a**) Representative en face images from a FRAP experiment on MP-GFP expressed olfactory cilia, depicting four epochs: pre-bleach, bleach, post-bleach, and post-recovery. The red rectangle denotes the photobleached area. Scale 10 μm. (**b**) Fluorescence intensity over time of the cilium that was bleached (denoted by arrow)

2 Materials

All solutions should be prepared with ultrapure water at room temperature. Reagents should be stored at room temperature unless noted.

2.1 Intranasal Viral Administration

1. Adult mice (*see* **Note 1**).
2. Adenovirus with construct of interest (1×10^{10} viral particles).
3. Anesthetic xylazine (100 mg/kg) and ketamine (10 mg/kg), or isoflurane and method of delivery (insulin syringe or vaporizer chamber, respectively).
4. Bleach solution: 10% bleach in water.

5. 70% ethanol.
6. Micropipettes and micropipette tips.
7. ABSL2 Biosafety Cabinet.

2.2 Dissection

1. Artificial cerebrospinal fluid (aCSF) solution: 124 mM NaCl, 3 mM KCl, 1.3 mM $MgSO_47H_2O$, 26 mM HCO_3, 1.25 mM NaH_2PO_4, 15 mM glucose, and 2 mM $CaCl_2$. Use a magnetic stir bar and stirring hot plate to mix the solution until solutes are dissolved. Sterilize with 0.22-micron filter apparatus. Store at 4 °C (*see* **Note 2**).
2. Straight point forceps.
3. Blunt point forceps.
4. Large, dissecting scissors (7″).
5. Small, curved scissor (4-½″).
6. Larger Petri dish (100 mm diameter).
7. Dissection Petri dish (50 mm diameter).
8. Disposable underpad.
9. Open diamond bath imaging chamber, referred to as imaging chamber (Warner instruments RC 26).
10. Slice holder (harp).
11. Upright light microscope.
12. Carbogen gas cylinder: 95% O_2, 5% CO_2.
13. CO_2 gas cylinder (100% CO_2).
14. Ice.
15. Ice bucket.
16. Aerator bubble diffuser.
17. Conical centrifuge tube (50 mL).

2.3 Confocal Microscopy and Analysis

1. Inverted confocal microscope with fluorescence imaging capability and oil immersion lens (e.g., laser scanning Nikon A1 inverted epifluorescence microscope with xenon lamp) for olfactory cilia imaging.
2. Inverted confocal microscope with TIRF (100× CFI APO TIRF 1.49 NA, 1.5× tube lens, ZT488/561rpc dichroic, ZET488/561x excitation filter, ZET488/561mTIRF emission filter).
3. EMCCD camera (iXon X3 DU897).
4. Immersion oil.
5. Software supplied by microscope manufacturer for imaging, for example, elements for Nikon systems.
6. ImageJ or Fiji for image reconstruction and analysis.

3 Methods

3.1 Intranasal Viral Delivery

The outlined procedure involves the viral delivery of fluorescent proteins; however, an alternative is the use of odorant receptor reporter mice though this approach limits labeling to a specific OSN subpopulation (*see* **Note 3**). See Table 1 for a list of published viral constructs that have been utilized to visualize olfactory cilia.

1. In an ABSL2 Biosafety Cabinet, anesthetize adult mice by either intraperitoneal injection of a cocktail of xylazine/ketamine or administration of isoflurane in an appropriate vaporizer chamber.
2. Aspirate the desired volume of virus (10–35 μL) using a micropipette.
3. When the mouse is adequately sedated, scruff and hold the mouse upright ensuring its arms and tail are held.
4. Deliver a ~3 μL drop of viral solution at the opening of the mouse's nostril (*see* **Note 4**).
5. Allow for the mouse to inhale the droplet and then place another drop of viral solution on the opposite nostril.

Table 1
Ciliary and transition zone proteins ectopically expressed in olfactory cilia

Category	Olfactory cilia protein or lipid	References
Inert ciliary markers	Myristoylation and palmitoylation (MyrPalm), dual palmitoylation (PalmPalm)	[23]
Ciliary transport and adaptor complexes	IFT(IFT122, IFT88), BBSome (BBS1-5,10)	[12, 13, 23]
Motor proteins	Kinesin (Kif17, Kap3a), Dynein (Dync2li1)	[12, 23]
Olfactory cascade components	ORs (M71-GFP, I7), AC3, CNG channel (CNGA2, CNGB1), Gαo	[11, 23, 26, 27]
Lipids	PI(3,4)P2 (PLCδ1-PH, Tapp1), PI4P (P4M-SidM), PIP3 (Btk), cholesterol (DH4), phosphatidylserine (Lact-C2), sphingomyelin (Eqt2-SM), glycosyl phosphatidylinositol (GPI)	[14]
Other ciliary proteins	ARL13B, alpha-tubulin, basal body (Centrin2), transition zone (NPHP4), proximal segment (Efhc1)	[13, 23, 26, 27]
Calcium probe	Calcium probe (GCaMP6f)	[14]
Probes to manipulate cilia	Inwardly rectifying potassium channel (Kir2.1), ORs (M71, I7, Olfr78)	[14, 28]

These proteins have all been utilized in publications to investigate cilia of olfactory sensory neurons. These ciliary proteins were tagged with fluorescent proteins in order to be visualized with fluorescence microscopy

6. Repeat **steps 4** and **5** until the desired volume has been delivered (*see* **Note 5**).
7. Place the mouse back in its cage and verify that the mouse recovers from the anesthesia (5–10 min).
8. Repeat **steps 1–7** for every mouse that will be intranasally administered viral solution.
9. Dispose of the micropipette tip and tube that contained viral solution in a 10% bleach solution.
10. Clean the surface of the biosafety cabinet with 70% ethanol.
11. Repeat administration of virus (**steps 1–10**) once daily for a total of 3 days (*see* **Note 6**).
12. Ten days after the third day of viral infection thus allowing for adequate protein expression, experiments can be performed (*see* **Note 7**).

3.2 Tissue Preparation

1. Place the bottle of aCSF into an ice bucket filled with ice.
2. Place the aerator bubble diffuser connected to the carbogen gas tank into the aCSF bottle and open the gas line.
3. Allow 15 min preceding tissue dissection for adequate aCSF aeration.
4. Lay out the disposable underpad where dissection will take place, preferably by the light upright microscope.
5. Euthanize the mouse with CO_2, or whichever method of euthanasia is approved by the user's IACUC protocol.
6. On the disposable underpad, decapitate the mouse using the larger scissors.
7. With the smaller scissors remove the skin and jaw from the mouse.
8. With blunt pointed forceps, remove the eyes and the soft palate.
9. On a large Petri dish, with a razor blade bisect the head along the cranial midline, using the sagittal suture connecting the parietal bones as guides.
10. Place one half of the snout, preferably the most intact, in a conical tube with freshly carbogenated aCSF that then should be closed and placed on ice for later use.
11. Place the other half of the snout in a dissection Petri dish and add aCSF until the tissue is fully submerged.
12. Under the light upright microscope, remove the septum and midline nasal bone from the snout.

13. Next, use the blunt point forceps to stabilize the snout and the straight point forceps to dissect out (remove) the olfactory turbinates (*see* **Note 8**).
14. With forceps, position the dissected turbinates onto the imaging chamber with the OE facing down.
15. With blunt point forceps, adjust the position of the turbinates as needed to ensure the surface of the OE lies flat.
16. Place the tissue holder on top of the tissue on the imaging chamber.
17. With a micropipette, add 300 μL of freshly carbogenated aCSF to the imaging chamber.

3.3 En Face Imaging

1. Prior to dissection, power on the xenon lamp, lasers, and the inverted confocal microscope.
2. Turn on the A1R box unit if conducting static or FRAP imaging. Power on the TIRF unit, and press the button for the desired laser wavelength if conducting TIRF imaging.
3. Power on the computer, and open the appropriate Nikon Elements software for the experiment of choice ("Nikon A1 Confocal" for the static condition and FRAP imaging or "Nikon TIRF" for TIRF imaging).
4. Once the Tissue Preparation (Subheading 3.2) steps have been completed, place the imaging chamber onto the inverted microscope stage so that the OE is facing the objective lens.
5. Using a low-magnification air interface lens (10× or 20×), locate regions of the OE that have fluorescing cilia.
6. Remove the imaging chamber, switch to a high-magnification lens (60× or 100×), and apply a droplet of the appropriate immersion oil (*see* **Note 9**).
7. Put the imaging chamber back on the stage, and identify a region of interest (ROI) with a low enough area of infection to resolve cilia from individual OSNs (*see* **Note 10**).
8. To establish the appropriate settings and collect images with the appropriate instructions, go to Subheading 3.3.1 for static conditions, Subheading 3.3.2 for TIRF, and Subheading 3.3.3 for FRAP microscopy.
9. Continue imaging cilia of OSNs in other regions in the OE (*see* **Note 11**).
10. Following, the second half of the snout that was preserved in aCSF on ice can now be dissected (repeat Subheading 3.2 Tissue Preparation **steps 12–17**) and imaged (repeat Subheading 3.3 En Face Imaging **steps 1–9**).

3.3.1 Static Condition Imaging

The following imaging method will result in confocal images of olfactory cilia under static conditions, meaning no dynamic processes or time-lapse images are recorded.

1. Under the "Acquisition" control panel, click the lasers that will be used (405, 488, 561, and/or 647 nm).
2. Set the appropriate pin hole size, which is typically 1.2 AU.
3. Set the scan size to 1024 × 1024 pixels, to set the resolution of the image.
4. Set the pixel dwell time to 2.2 frames/s.
5. Start scanning by pressing "live" and clicking "Remove Interlock."
6. Set the laser power ("Laser") to between 3% and 6%, detector sensitivity ("HV") between 50 and 100, and "Offset" to 0.

   Repeat this step for every laser.
7. Set the z-thickness to 0.5 μm.
8. Set the top and bottom z-position and obtain an image by hitting "Run now."
9. After obtaining an image, project the z-stack to maximum intensity. Then press the "Pixel Saturation Indication" button on the image to determine if there is saturation, meaning the signal is outside of the dynamic range. If the signal is too low or too high, adjust the laser power or detector sensitivity accordingly (*see* **Note 12**).
10. Continue searching for and imaging other regions by either using the eyepiece or scanning with the microscope system and repeating **steps 5** and **8** (*see* **Note 13**).

3.3.2 TIRF Imaging

Total internal reflection fluorescence (TIRF) microscopy can dramatically improve the signal-to-noise ratio and significantly reduce the photodamage to the tissue while maintaining high resolution of confocal imaging. Uniquely, TIRF imaging allows for the visualization of cellular dynamic events occurring near the plasma membrane. Therefore, certain ciliary proteins, especially those involved in the transport of cargo, namely, IFT and BBSome-related proteins, can be visualized utilizing TIRF imaging. The following procedure describes settings and the procedure for observing the movement of IFT88-GFP in the cilia of OSNs (Fig. 3):

1. Fill an empty imaging chamber with aCSF, and put the chamber on the objective for the laser alignment.
2. Power on the Perfect Focus System (PFS) controller to prevent drifting.
3. Press the Focus button (PFS-ON indicator) on the Front Operation Panel. Adjust the focus using the focus knob on

the microscope. The PFS-ON indicator stops blinking and lights up as green when the PFS has been initiated.

4. Once PFS is engaged, z-direction adjustment using the focus knob is disabled. Therefore, use the optional hand wheel to make fine adjustments in the z-direction.
5. Start live imaging (scanning).
6. On the TiPad under "Lamps," set the TIRF laser angle number to 3200 (*see* **Note 14**).
7. Use the adjustment screws to focus the laser. This is accomplished by visualizing the transmitted light pointed at the ceiling focusing by becoming as close to a point as possible (*see* **Note 15**).
8. Adjust the laser power based on the intensity of the fluorescence. Under AOTF Pad, select the desired laser wavelength and adjust the laser power to 10% (*see* **Note 16**).
9. To acquire a time series video, go to the menu bar and click "View," and select the "ND Stimulation" toolbox.
10. Check the "Save to File" checkbox to save the file while imaging.
11. Check the box labeled "Time" under the "Order of Experiment" heading. Then click on the button labeled "Add" under "Time schedule." Set "0 s" for Interval and "3 min" for Duration to get a zero delay interval TIRF time series.
12. Set the following camera settings under the "DU-897 Settings" panel: Auto Exposure, 200 ms; Readout Speed, 10 MHz; EM Gain Multiplier, 300; Conversion Gain, 2.4x.
13. Place the imaging chamber with the specimen onto the microscope stage for imaging (*see* **Note 17**).
14. Find an ROI either using eyepiece or scanning with the microscope system and click "Run now" in the ND Stimulation toolbox once ready for acquisition.
15. To obtain additional time series videos, go to another field of view, and repeat the previous step.

3.3.3 FRAP Imaging

To measure the rates of turnover or entrance of fluorescently tagged molecules in cilia, fluorescence recovery after photobleaching (FRAP) imaging can be utilized. FRAP takes advantage of the phenomena of high-intensity light denaturing fluorescent molecules leading to the loss of fluorescence. After photobleaching, the fluorescent signal is recorded over time, and the dynamics or mobility of the molecule can be measured based on the recovery rate of fluorescence. Here we use a Nikon A1 Confocal Microscope to perform FRAP microscopy on MP-GFP-labeled cilia of OSNs (Fig. 4) (*see* **Note 18**).

1. To set up the photobleaching parameters, on the menu bar click "View," then "Acquisition Controls," and select "A1plus Stimulation" to open the toolbox.
2. Within the A1plus Stimulation panel, up to three ROI settings (S1, S2, S3) can be assigned with different bleach laser powers. For every ROI to have the same photobleaching setting, check the box labeled "Synchronize lasers."
3. Select the desired laser to photobleach (488, 561, or 647 nm), and choose the power of stimulation for photobleaching. Typically, a laser power close to or equal to 100% is used for photobleaching. Set other lasers to 0%.
4. Set scan speed as 1 fps. Set the HV (detector sensitivity) as "Zero HV" (the standard setting).
5. The ND Stimulation panel is the control window to set time parameters. To open the toolbox, go to the menu bar and click "View," then click "Acquisition Controls," and select "ND Stimulation."
6. The FRAP experimental process should have at least three time phases: Acquisition, Bleaching, and Waiting.

Depending on the experimental need, the interval for acquisition or stimulation (time between image cycles) and number of loops for each phase can be changed (*see* **Note 19**).

1. Begin by setting up the acquisition phase by clicking on the button labeled "Add" under "Time schedule." Then under "Acq/Stim," choose "Acquisition." Set 3 s for "Interval," 20 s for "Duration," and 8 for "Loops."
2. To set up the bleaching phase, click on the button labeled "Add" under "Time schedule." Then under "Acq/Stim," choose "Bleaching," click "S1" for "ROIs." Set "No delay" for "Interval," 3 s for "Duration," and 3 for "Loops."
3. Set up the waiting phase by clicking on the button labeled "Add" under "Time schedule." Then under "Acq/Stim," choose "Waiting." Set 10 s for "Interval," 3 min for "Duration," and 20 for "Loops."
4. Check the button labeled "save to file." Under "Path" choose the folder where the file will be saved and set the filename.
5. Once these have been set, proceed with checking the "Perform Time Measurement" box. This is useful for seeing real-time fluorescent signal changes.
6. To set your ROI and prevent bleaching, click "capture" to obtain a static image. Then, on the right-hand side of the image, click the ROI tool. Choose the shape that best fits the experiment. The ideal geometric shape to photobleach olfactory cilia is a rectangle. Therefore, choose the "Draw

Rectangular ROI" to draw a rectangle over a single or multiple cilia in the stimulation ROI. The ROI can be moved, and the size is adjustable.

7. Right-click the selected ROI, and select "Use as Stimulation ROI: S1" to assign it the stimulation settings in **step 3**.
8. To be able to acquire images faster, use the Digital zoom function. Changing the scanning speed and the number of pixels per frame would allow you to set the time for acquisition and bleaching.
9. Click "Apply Stimulation Settings" when changes are made to the ROI position, ROI order, ROI designation, laser designation, or laser power, otherwise, the previous settings will be used.
10. Click "Run now" in the ND Stimulation toolbox to start the experiment.
11. Repeat **steps 12–16** to perform the FRAP experiment in another field of view.

3.4 Image Processing and Data Analysis

A common use of en face imaging under static conditions of the OE is for the analysis of ciliation of OSNs, namely, the number and length of the cilia on OSNs.

3.4.1 Static Condition Analysis

1. After opening the image file on ImageJ, stack the file by clicking "Image," then "Stack," then "Z Project…," and then input the start and stop slice, the projection type as "Max Intensity." and press "OK."
2. Use either the "Segmented Line" or "Freehand Line" tool on the main menu to draw the olfactory cilium from the tip to its base making sure to not draw into the dendritic knob and double click when done. Repeat this process until every discernable cilium on an individual OSN is analyzed (Fig. 2b).
3. Utilize the "Multi-point" tool to count the number of cilia on a given OSN.
4. Measure the ROIs created, and plot the average cilium length per OSN and the average number of cilia per OSN (Fig. 2c).

3.4.2 TIRF Analysis

The speed of the fluorescent protein of interest imaged during TIRF is measured by quantitatively analyzing kymographs. This procedure allows for the analysis of the linear motion of particle-like objects.

1. Begin by downloading the ImageJ plugin KymoResliceWide, StackReg, and TurboReg. Copy these folders into the folder entitled "Plugins" that is within the "ImageJ" folder on the computer.

2. Open the image file on ImageJ.
3. On the main menu click "Plugins" and then "StackReg." Run "Stackreg" to reduce/eliminate xy drift.
4. Access the "Segmented Line," adjust the thickness of the line to fit the diameter of the cilium (Edit > Option > Line Width), and draw a line across the olfactory cilium that is of interest for analysis from the tip to the base.
5. On the main menu, click "Plugins" and then "KymoReslice-Wide." Under the intensity click "Maximum" from the pull-down menu, and click the box for the option "Rotate 90 degrees." Make sure no other option is pressed. Finally, press "OK."
6. The kymograph plots the particle-like objects movements along the cilium with time on the x-axis and the distance on the y-axis.
7. To obtain the speed of particle motion, the kymograph is analyzed by first utilizing the "Straight Line" tool and drawing a line from left to right on the kymograph (Fig. 3b).
8. Use Image J- Analyze → Measure or press "M" key to measure angle θ. which is the angle of the path of the IFT train against the horizontal axis.
9. To convert the angle degree to radian, multiply the angle degree by $\pi/180$.
10. To get the velocity of particles in unit of pixel, the particle velocities were calculated as velocity = $\tan\theta$.

3.4.3 FRAP Analysis

1. Open the FRAP file on ImageJ.
2. To properly analyze the data, all the data must be internally normalized. To do so, utilize the rectangle tool to draw a "Rectangle ROI" in a region lacking fluorescence to collect background fluorescent intensities.
3. Use either the Segmented Line tool or Freehand Line to draw the olfactory cilium outside of the photobleaching region to serve as the reference. Continue the process for every olfactory cilium within the photobleached region.
4. Select "Plot Z-axis Profile" in Fiji (Image → Stacks → Plot Z-axis Profile), and the extracted fluorescent intensity values can be measured from this window.
5. Subtract the background fluorescent intensities, then the FRAP data of each cilium can be plotted using GraphPad Prism (Fig. 4b).

4 Notes

1. The outlined intranasal viral delivery is for adult mice. We have previously described a procedure for young mice as well as rats [25], which are also amenable to viral delivery of fluorescent proteins coupled with en face imaging for assessment of olfactory cilia.
2. For long-term storage of aCSF (longer than 2 weeks), do not include $CaCl_2$ as it will precipitate out of solution or glucose which causes bacterial growth.
3. Though limiting, in lieu of virally delivering fluorescent proteins, odorant receptor fluorescent reporter mice are available at the Jackson Laboratory and can be utilized for the method. The following are the various murine model lines and stock numbers: M71-IRES-tau-GFP (006676), M72-IRES-tau-GFP (006678), M72-IRES- tauCherry (029637), SR1-IRES-tau-GFP (006717), MOR23-IRES-tau-GFP (006643), Olfr151- IRES-tau-mCherry (0294290), and OR1A1-IRES-tau-mCherry (029600).
4. When delivering virus to the mouse, ensure that the micropipette does not come in contact with the phylum to prevent harm.
5. Allow enough time for the mouse to properly be sedated to avoid it regaining consciousness during the viral administration. However, it is important if using an isoflurane chamber that the mouse is not in the chamber for an excessive time as this will result in death.
6. Administration of virus at a titer of for 3 days leads to an infection rate of about 15% of neurons [13] and is optimal for en face imaging of cilia from individual OSNs.
7. Though the optimal time after infection to conduct en face imaging is 10 days after adenovirus delivery, fluorescence is initially visible at 24 h after infection, and experiments may be conducted then. This time frame may also be dependent on the promoter of the viral construct. This procedure utilizes adenovirus serotype 5, and the construct has a CMV promoter.
8. During dissection the user can either remove all of the turbinates or individual turbinates or store the others in ice-cold aerated aCSF.
9. Ensure that the objective lens is away from the top of the stage (hit escape on the microscope) and that there is sufficient oil on the surface of the lens. This could help protect the lens from damage.

10. Viral infection with adenovirus will predominantly infect OSNs but can also infect the supportive cells, sustentacular cells [12, 13]. Sustentacular cells are microvillar and reside below the ciliary layer of OSNs. Both the difference in location and morphology of the cilia on OSNs compared to the microvilli on sustentacular cells make it easy to delineate one from the other.
11. The tissue in aCSF remains healthy for about an hour at room temperature. Both the deterioration of the health of the tissue and a defective preparation/dissection (cilia are fragile and if not careful forceps can break the cilia) of the tissue are evident by fragments of broken off cilia.
12. It is important to note that changing the scan size, pixel dwell, or pin hole will all require the adjustment of the laser settings.
13. Do not change the imaging parameters except for setting the top and bottom z-position as the tissue may be uneven. Keeping the settings standard within an experiment is imperative for proper analysis of data, especially if assessing pixel intensity.
14. A 3200 number is the angle where the TIRF laser is perfectly straight; however, further adjustment may be needed.
15. The visible light on the ceiling should be a point. If it is not a point but instead a vertical or horizontal line, adjust the focus using adjustment screws.
16. Make sure that the TIRF laser settings illuminate the tissue enough for visualization during image acquisition but are not too intense as this will accelerate bleaching of the sample.
17. Use 100 ms exposure to search for OSNs to avoid photobleaching. Once the target OSN is found, change exposure to 200 ms.
18. The outlined procedure uses the A1 Nikon system; however, other inverted confocal microscopes can be substituted. The user can ask the manufacturer's representatives for assistance or reference the manual to adjust the setting based on the microscope.
19. For FRAP experiments, long delays may protect the entire sample from photobleaching. However, if the fluorescently tagged protein's movement is rapid, then no or a short delay is better. If the protein dynamics are extremely slow, a much longer delay is needed.

Acknowledgments

We acknowledge Dr. Kirill Ukhanov for providing a representative whole-mount staining image and technical assistance. We thank Dr. Cedric Uytingco for providing a representative TIRF image. This work was supported by the National Institute of Deafness and Other Communication Disorders R01DC019345 (JRM), T32DC015994 (JCH), and F31DC020638 (JCH).

References

1. Bloom G (1954) Studies on the olfactory epithelium of the frog and the toad with the aid of light and electron microscopy. Z Zellforsch Mikrosk Anat 41(1):89–100. https://doi.org/10.1007/BF00340285
2. Menco BP, Farbman AI (1985) Genesis of cilia and microvilli of rat nasal epithelia during pre-natal development. I. Olfactory epithelium, qualitative studies. J Cell Sci 78:283–310
3. Menco BP, Farbman AI (1985) Genesis of cilia and microvilli of rat nasal epithelia during pre-natal development. II. Olfactory epithelium, a morphometric analysis. J Cell Sci 78: 311–336
4. Okano M, Weber AF, Frommes SP (1967) Electron microscopic studies on the distal border of the canine olfactory epithelium. J Ultrastruct Res 17(5):487–502. https://doi.org/10.1016/s0022-5320(67)80137-0
5. Kavoi B, Makanya A, Hassanali J, Carlsson HE, Kiama S (2010) Comparative functional structure of the olfactory mucosa in the domestic dog and sheep. Ann Anat 192(5):329–337. https://doi.org/10.1016/j.aanat.2010.07.004
6. Kratzing JE (1975) The fine structure of the olfactory and vomeronasal organs of a lizard (Tiliqua scincoides scincoides). Cell Tissue Res 156(2):239–252. https://doi.org/10.1007/BF00221807
7. Hansen A (2007) Olfactory and solitary chemosensory cells: two different chemosensory systems in the nasal cavity of the American alligator, Alligator mississippiensis. BMC Neurosci 8:64. https://doi.org/10.1186/1471-2202-8-64
8. Schulte E, Holl A (1971) Ultrastructure of the olfactory epithelium of *Calamoichthys calabaricus* J. A. Smoth (Pisces, Brachiopterygii). Z Zellforsch Mikrosk Anat 120(2):261–279. https://doi.org/10.1007/BF00335539
9. Hansen A, Zielinski BS (2005) Diversity in the olfactory epithelium of bony fishes: development, lamellar arrangement, sensory neuron cell types and transduction components. J Neurocytol 34(3–5):183–208. https://doi.org/10.1007/s11068-005-8353-1
10. Green WW, Uytingco CR, Ukhanov K, Kolb Z, Moretta J, McIntyre JC et al (2018) Peripheral gene therapeutic rescue of an olfactory ciliopathy restores sensory input, axonal pathfinding, and odor-guided behavior. J Neurosci 38(34): 7462–7475. https://doi.org/10.1523/JNEUROSCI.0084-18.2018
11. Uytingco CR, Williams CL, Xie C, Shively DT, Green WW, Ukhanov K et al (2019) BBS4 is required for intraflagellar transport coordination and basal body number in mammalian olfactory cilia. J Cell Sci 132(5). https://doi.org/10.1242/jcs.222331
12. Williams CL, Uytingco CR, Green WW, McIntyre JC, Ukhanov K, Zimmerman AD et al (2017) Gene therapeutic reversal of peripheral olfactory impairment in Bardet-Biedl syndrome. Mol Ther 25(4):904–916. https://doi.org/10.1016/j.ymthe.2017.02.006
13. McIntyre JC, Davis EE, Joiner A, Williams CL, Tsai IC, Jenkins PM et al (2012) Gene therapy rescues cilia defects and restores olfactory function in a mammalian ciliopathy model. Nat Med 18(9):1423–1428. https://doi.org/10.1038/nm.2860
14. Ukhanov K, Uytingco C, Green W, Zhang L, Schurmans S, Martens JR (2022) INPP5E controls ciliary localization of phospholipids and the odor response in olfactory sensory neurons. J Cell Sci 135(5). https://doi.org/10.1242/jcs.258364
15. Xie C, Habif JC, Uytingco CR, Ukhanov K, Zhang L, de Celis C et al (2021) Gene therapy rescues olfactory perception in a clinically relevant ciliopathy model of Bardet-Biedl syndrome. FASEB J 35(9):e21766. https://doi.org/10.1096/fj.202100627R
16. Oberland S, Neuhaus EM (2014) Whole mount labeling of cilia in the main olfactory system of mice. J Vis Exp 94. https://doi.org/10.3791/52299

17. Alevra M, Schwartz P, Schild D (2012) Direct measurement of diffusion in olfactory cilia using a modified FRAP approach. PLoS One 7(7):e39628. https://doi.org/10.1371/journal.pone.0039628
18. Jenkins PM, Hurd TW, Zhang L, McEwen DP, Brown RL, Margolis B et al (2006) Ciliary targeting of olfactory CNG channels requires the CNGB1b subunit and the kinesin-2 motor protein, KIF17. Curr Biol 16(12):1211–1216. https://doi.org/10.1016/j.cub.2006.04.034
19. Delling M, DeCaen PG, Doerner JF, Febvay S, Clapham DE (2013) Primary cilia are specialized calcium signalling organelles. Nature 504(7479):311–314. https://doi.org/10.1038/nature12833
20. Fan S, Fogg V, Wang Q, Chen XW, Liu CJ, Margolis B (2007) A novel Crumbs3 isoform regulates cell division and ciliogenesis via importin beta interactions. J Cell Biol 178(3):387–398. https://doi.org/10.1083/jcb.200609096
21. Hansen JN, Kaiser F, Klausen C, Stüven B, Chong R, Bönigk W et al (2020) Nanobody-directed targeting of optogenetic tools to study signaling in the primary cilium. elife 9. https://doi.org/10.7554/eLife.57907
22. Iwadate Y (2003) Photolysis of caged calcium in cilia induces ciliary reversal in *Paramecium caudatum*. J Exp Biol 206(Pt 7):1163–1170. https://doi.org/10.1242/jeb.00219
23. Williams CL, McIntyre JC, Norris SR, Jenkins PM, Zhang L, Pei Q et al (2014) Direct evidence for BBSome-associated intraflagellar transport reveals distinct properties of native mammalian cilia. Nat Commun 5:5813. https://doi.org/10.1038/ncomms6813
24. Xie C, Habif JC, Ukhanov K, Uytingco CR, Zhang L, Campbell RJ et al (2022) Reversal of ciliary mechanisms of disassembly rescues olfactory dysfunction in ciliopathies. JCI Insight. https://doi.org/10.1172/jci.insight.158736
25. Uytingco CR, Martens JR (2019) Intranasal delivery of adenoviral and AAV vectors for transduction of the mammalian peripheral olfactory system. Methods Mol Biol 1950:283–297. https://doi.org/10.1007/978-1-4939-9139-6_17
26. Corey EA, Ukhanov K, Bobkov YV, McIntyre JC, Martens JR, Ache BW (2021) Inhibitory signaling in mammalian olfactory transduction potentially mediated by Gα. Mol Cell Neurosci 110:103585. https://doi.org/10.1016/j.mcn.2020.103585
27. McIntyre JC, Joiner AM, Zhang L, Iñiguez-Lluhí J, Martens JR (2015) SUMOylation regulates ciliary localization of olfactory signaling proteins. J Cell Sci 128(10):1934–1945. https://doi.org/10.1242/jcs.164673
28. Zhao H, Ivic L, Otaki JM, Hashimoto M, Mikoshiba K, Firestein S (1998) Functional expression of a mammalian odorant receptor. Science 279(5348):237–242. https://doi.org/10.1126/science.279.5348.237

Chapter 2

Genome-Wide RNA Tomography in the Mouse Whole Olfactory Mucosa

Eman Abou Moussa, Melanie Makhlouf, Lisa S. Mathew, and Luis R. Saraiva

Abstract

Spatial transcriptomics allows for the genome-wide profiling of topographic gene expression patterns within a tissue of interest. Here, we describe our methodology to generate high-quality RNA-seq libraries from cryosections from fresh frozen mouse whole olfactory mucosae. This methodology can be extended to virtually any vertebrate organ or tissue sample.

Key words Spatial transcriptomics, RNA-sequencing, Tomo-seq, Low-input RNA, Cryosectioning, Whole olfactory mucosa, Olfaction

1 Introduction

The neuroepithelium of the mousewhole olfactory mucosa (WOM) is populated by ±10 million olfactory sensory neurons (OSNs), each expressing a single allele of an intact olfactory receptor (OR) [1]. In the last three decades, many researchers have tried to unravel the diversity and topographic organization of OSNs with techniques ranging from in situ hybridization to genome-wide RNA-sequencing (RNA-seq) methods [2–12].

The advent of spatial transcriptomics techniques allowed us to circumvent many of the technical limitations imposed by the conventional techniques mentioned above [13]. In this context, we recently applied a modified version of the original RNA-seq tomography (Tomo-seq) protocol [14] to the mouseWOM [15]. The technique involves the serial histological cryosectioning of fresh frozen mouseWOM samples along three Cartesian axes, followed by the RNA extractions of each cryosection, cDNA generation, preparation of low-input library RNA-seq preparation, and, finally, high-throughput sequencing.

Bradley J. Goldstein and Hiroaki Matsunami (eds.), *The Olfactory System*, Methods in Molecular Biology, vol. 2710, https://doi.org/10.1007/978-1-0716-3425-7_2,

In this chapter, we describe the methodology we use to generate high-quality RNA-seq libraries from cryosections of fresh frozen WOMmouse samples. Importantly, the protocol highlighted here can easily be extended to other tissues or organs from any vertebrate species. Indeed, we have successfully applied it on other fresh frozen mouse samples, such as the tibia bones and small intestines (unpublished data).

2 Materials

2.1 WOM Dissection and Cryosection

1. Dissection tools as needed (forceps, scissors, scalpels).
2. Peel-A-Way™ embedding mold (e.g., Merck, Catalog number: E6032).
3. Tissue-Tek® O.C.T. Compound.
4. Cryostat.
5. Microscopic slides.
6. RLT buffer (Qiagen, Catalog number: 79216) complemented with β-mercaptoethanol.

2.2 RNA Extraction from WOM Cryosections

RNeasy® Plus Mini Kit (Qiagen, Catalog number: 74104);

RLT Plus lysis buffer: 10 μl of β-mercaptoethanol (β-ME) per 1 ml of Buffer RLT Plus before use (*see* **Note 1**).

RNAse free DNAse Set (Qiagen, Catalog number: 79254);

RNAse free DNAse Mix: prepare freshly by adding 6 μl of DNAse I to 44 μl of RDD buffer in a total of 50 μl for each sample.

1. DNAse I mix.
2. Agilent RNA 6000 Pico Kit.
3. Bioanalyzer 2100 system.

2.3 cDNA Synthesis and Amplification and RNA-seq Library Preparation

1. SMART-Seq® v4 Ultra® Low Input RNA Kit v4 for Sequencing (TakaraBio, Cat# 634891) (*see* **Note 2**).
   (a) Lysis Mix A (for eight reactions): 10X lysis buffer 1.6 μl; 40 U/μl RNase inhibitor 0.5 μl; H_2O 6.9 μl; 12 μM 3' SMART CDS Primer II A 7 μl.
   (b) RT Mix B (for eight reactions): 5x Ultra Low First-Strand Buffer 3 μl; 48 μMSMART-Seq v4 Oligo 0.5 μl; 40 U/μl RNase Inhibitor 1.5 μl; H2O 8.5 μl; SMARTScribe RT 8 μl.
   (c) PCR Mix C (for eight reactions): 2x SeqAmp PCR Buffer 40 μl; 12 μM PCR Primer II A – v4 4 μl; SeqAmp DNA Polymerase 8 μl; H_2O 24 μl.
2. PCR thermal cycler.

3. Nuclease-free water.
4. Freshly prepared 80% ethanol.
5. Magnetic separation rack.
6. Ampure XP Reagent for PCR purification (Beckman Coulter, Cat# A63880).
7. Qubit dsDNA High Sensitivity Assay Kit (Invitrogen).
8. Agilent High Sensitivity DNA Kit.
9. Perkin Elmer GXII.
10. Quant-iT dsDNA High Sensitivity Assay (Thermo Fisher).
11. FlexStation 3 (Molecular Devices, USA).
12. Nextera XT DNA Library Preparation Kit (Illumina, Catalog number: 15032354) (*see* **Note 3**). cDNA Tagmentation Mix (per reaction): Tagmentation DNA Buffer 5 μl; Amplification Tagmentation Mix 2.5 μl.
13. Nextera XT Index Kit V2 (Illumina, Catalog number: 15052163).

3 Methods

The protocol is divided into several steps, which could be paused at specific time points and resumed at a later point. The first step involves dissecting, embedding, and freezing the WOM. The second step involves the serial cryosectioning (35 μm) of the WOM along one of the three Cartesian axes. The third step includes RNA extraction from individual cryosections. The fourth step entails cDNA preparation, followed by purification and cleanup using magnetic beads. Finally, RNA-sequencing libraries are generated using a modified purified using magnetic beads.

3.1 WOM Dissection and Cryosection

1. Carefully dissect the WOM of each mouse, making sure to remove all the surrounding glands, bone, and cartilage without damaging the WOM (*see* **Note 4**).
2. Fill the cubes with the Tissue-Tek® O.C.T. Compound to the upper edge, avoid making bubbles (turn the closed bottle upside down for some seconds, then open it in the same position and fill the cubes). Embed the dissected WOMs in OCT aligning them in the desired orientation (*see* **Note 5**), and immediately freeze them using dry ice or liquid nitrogen.
3. Each WOM is cryosectioned along each of the three Cartesian axes: dorsal-ventral (DV, N = 3), anterior-posterior (AP, N = 3), or lateral-medial-lateral (LML, N = 3). The first and every other cryosection (35 μm thick) is collected to a microscopy slide to keep a visual record of the tissue structure.

The second and every other cryosection (35 μm thick) is collected into 1.5 mL Eppendorf tubes containing 350 μl RLT Plus Buffer supplemented with 1% 2-mercaptoethanol, immediately frozen in dry ice and kept at −80 °C until extraction (*see* **Note 6**).

3.2 RNA Extraction from WOM Cryosections

1. Transfer the homogenized lysate (350 μl) to a Qiagen gDNA Eliminator spin column in a 2 ml collection tube.
2. Centrifuge for 1 min at ≥8000 g (≥10,000 rpm). Discard the column and save the flow-through. Add 1 volume (usually 350 μl) of freshly prepared 70% ethanol to the flow-through to precipitate RNA, and mix well by gentle pipetting. Do not centrifuge. Proceed immediately to step 4.
3. Transfer up to 700 μl of the sample, including any precipitate, to a RNeasy spin column placed in a 2 ml collection tube (supplied, stored in the 4°fridge). Close the lid and centrifuge for 1 min at ≥8000 g. Discard the flow-through.
4. Add 350 μl Buffer RW1 to the RNeasy Mini spin column (in a 2 ml collection tube). Close the lid and centrifuge for 1 min at ≥8000 g. Discard the flow-through.
5. Add 50 μl of RNAse-free DNAse mix (*see* **Note 7**) in the middle of the column without touching the column membrane. Close the lid and incubate for 30 min at room temperature.
6. Add 350 μl Buffer RW1 to the RNeasy Mini spin column. Close the lid and centrifuge for 1 min at ≥8000 g. Discard the flow-through.
7. Add 500 μl Buffer RPE (Buffer RPE is prepared by adding 44 ml of 100% ethanol to the supplied Buffer RPE bottle) to the RNeasy spin column. Close the lid and centrifuge for 2 min at ≥8000 g. Discard the flow-through.
8. Add 500 μl 80% ethanol (freshly prepared) to the RNeasy spin column. Close the lid gently, and centrifuge for 2 min at ≥8000 g (≥10,000 rpm) to wash the spin column membrane. Discard the collection tube with the flow-through.
9. Place the RNeasy spin column in a new 2 ml collection tube. Centrifuge at full speed for 3 min to dry the membrane. Discard the collection tube with the flow-through.
10. Place the RNeasy spin column in a new 1.5 ml collection tube (supplied). Add 14 μl RNase-free water directly to the spin column membrane. Close the lid and centrifuge for 1 min at ≥8000 g to elute the RNA. Repeat the elution by re-dispensing RNA eluate into the RNeasy spin column and centrifuge for an additional 1 min.

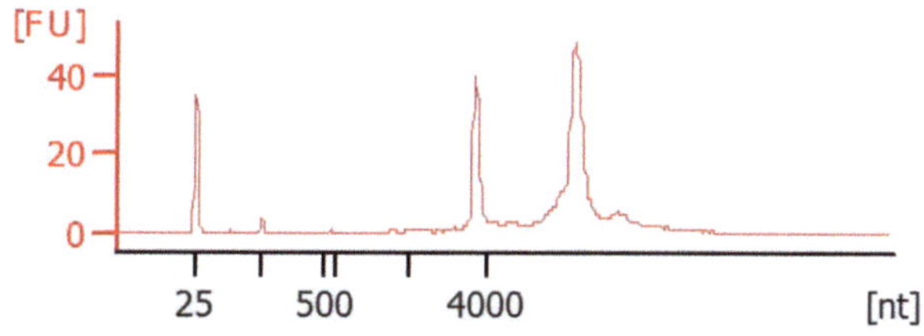

Fig. 1 Representative example of an electropherogram of RNA extracted from a cryosection using this protocol showing high-quality RNA. This sample has an RNA Integrity Number (RIN) of 9.9 (on a scale ranging from 0 to 10, where 10 is the highest quality number). FU – fluorescence units

11. Discard the RNeasy spin column. Take 1 μl of extracted RNA for quantification and quality check (place it on ice and see next step), and store the remaining extracted RNA at −80 °C for future applications.
12. Check the quantity and quality of the RNA by using the Agilent RNA 6000 Pico Kit on a Bioanalyzer 2100 system (see Fig. 1).

3.3 cDNA Synthesis and Amplification

1. On ice, mix 1.5 μl of Lysis Mix A with 2 μl of the cryosection RNA (avoid bubbles!). Place the PCR tubes (or the 96-well plate) in the thermocycler, and run the following program:
   (a) 72 °C for 3 min.
   (b) 4 °C for 10 min.
   (c) 25 °C for 1 min.
   (d) 4 °C on hold.
2. On ice, add 3.5 μl of RT Mix B to each tube (already containing 1.5 μl Lysis Mix A + 2 μl RNA). Place the PCR tubes or the 96-well plate in the thermocycler and run the following program:
   (a) 42 °C for 90 min.
   (b) 70 °C for 10 min.
   (c) 4 °C on hold.
3. On ice, add 1.5 μl of the mix from the previous step to 9 μl of PCR Reaction Mix C in new PCR tubes (or a new 96-well plate). Place the PCR tubes or the 96-well plate in the thermocycler and run the following program:
   (a) 95 °C for 1 min.
   (b) 21 cycles of:
      (i) 98 °C for 20 s.
      (ii) 65 °C, for 20 s.
      (iii) 68 °C for 5 min.

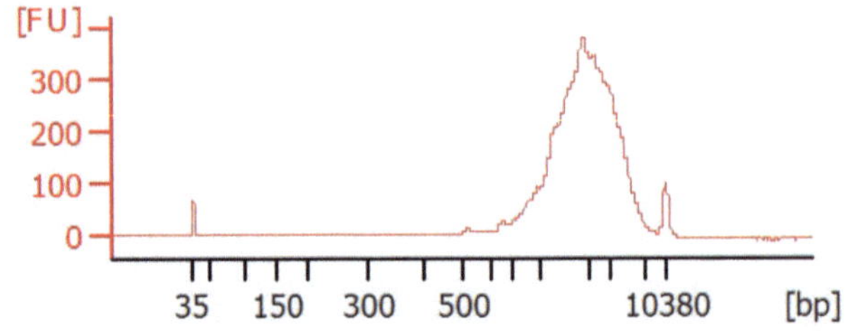

Fig. 2 Representative example of an electropherogram of cDNA generated using SMART-Seq® v4 Ultra® Low Input RNA Kit and quantified by Bioanalyzer 2100 system and Agilent High Sensitivity DNA Kit. FU, fluorescence units

(c) 72 °C for 10 m.

(d) 4 °C on hold.

4. Check the quantity and quality of the DNA by using the Agilent DNA High Sensitivity Kit on a Bioanalyzer 2100 system (Fig. 2).
5. Add 20 μl nuclease-free water to the sample plate, post-cDNA amplification to bring the total volume to 30 μl.
6. Add 30 μl (1X) of Ampure XP Reagent to each sample (*see* **Note 8**). Mix thoroughly by vortexing for 3–5 s or pipetting the entire volume up and down at least ten times (avoid bubbles and do a quick spin down if needed).
7. Incubate the beads-cDNA mixture at room temperature for 8 min to let the cDNA bind to the beads.
8. Briefly spin down the samples to collect the liquid from the side of the tubes or plate wells.
9. Place the samples on a magnetic separation plate for ~5 min or longer, until the liquid appears completely clear.
10. Remove and discard the supernatant taking care not to disturb the beads. Keep the samples on the magnet.
11. Add 200 μl of freshly made 80% ethanol to each sample and incubate for 30 s. Then, carefully remove and discard the supernatant, taking care not to disturb the beads. The cDNA remains bound to the beads during the washing process.
12. Repeat the 80% ethanol wash step.
13. Briefly centrifuge the samples to collect the liquid from the side of the tubes or plate wells.
14. Samples back on the magnet and remove any residual ethanol with a 20 μl pipette.
15. Be sure to dry the pellet only until it is just dry (*see* **Note 9**).
16. Once the beads are dry, remove the samples from the magnetic separation device and add 15 μl of elution buffer to the bead pellet. Mix thoroughly by pipetting or gently vortexing to resuspend the beads.

17. Incubate at room temperature for 2 min to rehydrate.
18. Briefly spin the samples to collect the liquid from the side of the tubes or plate wells. Place the samples back on the magnetic separation device for 1 min (or until the solution is completely clear).
19. Transfer clear supernatant (~13 μl) containing purified cDNA from each well to a new plate. Samples can be used in the next steps or stored at −20 °C.
20. Aliquot 1 μl of the amplified cDNA with 19 μl of nuclease-free water for validation on the Perkin Elmer GXII using the DNA High Sensitivity Assay. Successful cDNA synthesis and amplification should yield a distinct peak spanning 400 bp to 10,000 bp.
21. To ensure accurate input of 300 pg cDNA for downstream library preparation using the Illumina Nextera XT kit, 1 ul of cDNA is quantified using the Quant-iT dsDNA High Sensitivity Assay on the FlexStation 3 platform.

3.4 Preparation of RNA-Sequencing Libraries

Before constructing Nextera XT libraries, dilute all cDNA to the concentration of ~300 pg of cDNA/μl of H2O, as this is the ideal concentration according to the kit manufacturer.

1. Mix 1–2 μl of cDNA with 7.5 μl of the cDNA Tagmentation Mix.
2. Seal tube or plate, vortex at medium speed for 20 s, and centrifuge at 4000 rpm for 5 min to remove bubbles. Place the PCR tubes (or the 96-well plate) in the thermocycler and run the following program:
   (a) 55 °C for 10 min.
   (b) 10 °C hold.
3. On ice, add 2.5 μl of the neutralization NT buffer to each PCR tube/well from the previous step.
4. Seal tube or plate, vortex at medium speed for 20 s, and centrifuge at 4000 rpm for 5 min to remove bubbles.
5. On ice, add 7.5 μl of the NPM PCR Mix to each tube/well [containing 12 μl volume from the previous steps].
6. To the mix of the previous step, add 1.25 μl of Index Primer 1 (N7XX-N7XX) to each tube/well (*see* **Note 10**).
7. To the mix of the previous step, add 1.25 μl of Index Primer 2 (N5XX-N5XX) to each tube/well (*see* **Note 10**).
8. Seal the tube or plate, vortex at medium speed for 20 s, and centrifuge at 4000 rpm for 2 min to remove bubbles. Place the PCR tubes (or the 96-well plate) in the thermocycler and run the following program:

Table 1
Guide for sample pooling for RNA-seq library preparation

Number samples to be pooled	Volume per sample (μl)	Total pool volume (μl)	AMPure XP reagent volume (μl)
8	3	24	21.6
12	2	24	21.6
16	2	32	28.8
24	1	24	21.6
32	1	32	28.8
48	1	48	43.2
96	1	96	86.4

(a) 72 °C for 3 min.

(b) 95 °C for 30 s.

(c) 12 cycles of:

(i) 95 °C for 10 s.

(ii) 55 °C for 30 s.

(iii) 72 °C for 1 min.

(d) 72 °C for 5 min.

(e) 4 °C on hold.

9. To the pooled library, add the required amount of AMPure XP reagent (80% of the original volume), as listed in the Table 1 (*see* **Note 11**).
10. Mix well by pipetting up and down five times and incubate the bead mix at room temperature for 5 min.
11. Place the tube in the magnetic stand for 2 min.
12. Carefully remove the supernatant without disturbing the beads.
13. Add 180 μl of freshly prepared 70% ethanol, and incubate for 30 s on the magnetic stand, and remove the ethanol.
14. Carefully remove the supernatant without disturbing the beads.
15. Add 180 μl of freshly prepared 70% ethanol, and incubate for 30 s on the magnetic stand and remove the ethanol.
16. Allow the beads to air dry on the bench for 10–15 min (*see* **Note 12**).
17. Elute the samples by adding the required volume of DNA Suspension Buffer to its original volume (see table above).

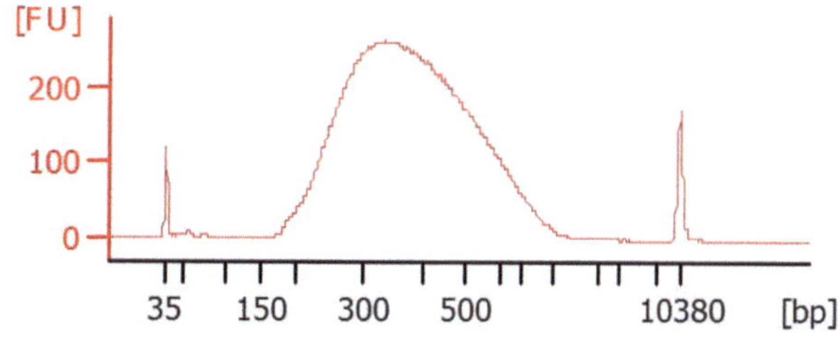

Fig. 3 Representative example of an electropherogram of a purified pooled Nextera XT Library and quantified using Bioanalyzer 2100 system and Agilent High Sensitivity DNA Kit. FU, fluorescence units

18. Vortex and incubate the tube for 2 min at room temperature.
19. Plate the tube on a magnetic stand for 2 min.
20. Transfer the entire volume of supernatant to another PCR tube.
21. Check the quantity and quality of the DNA by using the Agilent DNA High Sensitivity Kit on a Bioanalyzer 2100 system (Fig. 3).
22. Submit libraries for sequencing in an Illumina platform.

4 Notes

1. Prepare this buffer ahead of the collection of the cryosections. Note that Buffer RLT Plus containing β-ME can be stored at room temperature for up to 1 month.
2. Prepare and handle the Lysis Mix A, RT Mix B. and PCR Mix C on ice. Also, due to the low volumes per reaction, we recommend preparing each master mix for at least eight reactions. Ensure to scale up or down to the total number of desired reactions.
3. Prepare the cDNA Tagmentation Mix on ice, and immediately before using it. Ensure to scale up to the total number of desired reactions.
4. Removing all undesired tissue surrounding the WOM is a crucial step, as the transcripts present in it will contaminate the RNA isolated from the WOM.
5. Follow these instructions to align the WOM in the following orientations:
   (a) Dorsal–ventral (horizontal embedding): Place WOM horizontally with the dorsal side facing the bottom of the cube. Hold it with tweezers in a straight position, place it on dry ice, and keep holding WOM straight until the

OCT embedding solution freezes (it will become opaque white and solid).

(b) Lateral–medial–lateral (horizontal embedding): Place WOM horizontally with one of the lateral sides facing the bottom of the cube, parallel to the bottom of the cube. Hold it with tweezers in a straight position, place it on dry ice and keep holding WOM straight until the OCT embedding solution freezes (it will become opaque white and solid).

(c) Anterior–posterior (vertical embedding): Hold WOM vertically, parallel to the bottom of the cube, with the tip of the nose facing upwards and the part that contacted the olfactory bulb facing the bottom of the cub. Hold it with tweezers in a straight position, place it on dry ice, and keep holding WOM straight until the OCT embedding solution freezes (it will become opaque white and solid).

(d) If you are not planning to proceed directly to the next step, store the samples in the −80 °C freezer until future use.

6. Carefully drop each cryosection directly in the middle of a 1.5 ml Eppendorf tube containing 350 μl of pre-prepared RLT Plus lysis buffer. Make sure not to touch the walls of the tube and vortex for at least 10 sec to ensure the cryosection is completely dissolved and do a quick spin down if needed. RNA extraction can be performed immediately after this step. Alternatively, the samples can be temporarily stored in the cryo-chamber of the cryostat until a complete WOM is cryosectioned and then moved to the −20 °C freezer for longer-term storage. If the sample is to be processed after a freezing cycle, allow the sample to thaw at 4 °C and to equilibrate to room temperature before using it. After this, vortex each sample for 10 s before starting RNA extraction. Do a quick spin down if needed.

7. The RNAse free DNAse Set (Qiagen, Cat# 79254) is not provided with the RNeasy® Plus Mini Kit (Qiagen, Cat#74104) and should be ordered separately.

8. Before use, remove the Ampure XP Reagent from the 4 °C, and leave it at room temperature for 30 min. Prepare fresh 80% ethanol for the wash step.

9. If you over-dry the pellet, you will see visible cracks splitting it, and it will take longer than 2 min to rehydrate. If you under-dry the pellet, ethanol will remain in the sample wells. In both these cases, the recovery rate and yield of amplified cDNA will diminish.

10. Please read the “Index Adapters Pooling Guide” that comes with this product before deciding on which primer

combinations to use. Make sure to follow the guidelines for preparing libraries with balanced index combinations for sequencing on Illumina systems.

11. Before use, remove the Ampure XP Reagent from the 4 °C, and leave it at room temperature for 30 min. Prepare fresh 80% ethanol for the wash step. When pooling samples (see Table 1), work with volumes of at least 24 μl!
12. If you over-dry the pellet, you will see visible cracks splitting it, and it will take longer than 2 min to rehydrate. If you under-dry the pellet, ethanol will remain in the sample wells. In both these cases, the recovery rate and yield of amplified cDNA will diminish.

Acknowledgments

We want to thank the Integrated Genomic Services of Sidra Medicine for the technical support. This work was supported by Sidra Medicine (grant SDR400040 to L.R.S.) – a member of Qatar Foundation.

References

1. Kurian SM, Naressi RG, Manoel D, Barwich AS, Malnic B, Saraiva LR (2021) Odor coding in the mammalian olfactory epithelium. Cell Tissue Res 383:445–456
2. Ressler KJ, Sullivan SL, Buck LB (1993) *A* zonal organization of odorant receptor gene expression in the olfactory epithelium. Cell 73(3):597–609
3. Vassar R, Ngai J, Axel R (1993) Spatial segregation of odorant receptor expression in the mammalian olfactory epithelium. Cell 74(2): 309–318
4. Strotmann J, Wanner I, Krieger J, Raming K, Breer H (1992) Expression of odorant receptors in spatially restricted subsets of chemosensory neurones. Neuroreport 3:1053–1056
5. Miyamichi K, Serizawa S, Kimura HM, Sakano H (2005) Continuous and overlapping expression domains of odorant receptor genes in the olfactory epithelium determine the dorsal/ventral positioning of glomeruli in the olfactory bulb. J Neurosci 25:3586–3592
6. Zapiec B, Mombaerts P (2020) The zonal organization of odorant receptor gene choice in the main olfactory epithelium of the mouse. Cell Rep 30(12):4220–4234 e5
7. Saraiva LR, Riveros-McKay F, Mezzavilla M, Abou-Moussa EH, Arayata CJ, Makhlouf M, Trimmer C, Ibarra-Soria X, Khan M, Van Gerven L et al (2019) A transcriptomic atlas of mammalian olfactory mucosae reveals an evolutionary influence on food odor detection in humans. Sci Adv 5:eaax0396
8. Ibarra-Soria X, Nakahara TS, Lilue J, Jiang Y, Trimmer C, Souza MA, Netto PH, Ikegami K, Murphy NR, Kusma M et al (2017) Variation in olfactory neuron repertoires is genetically controlled and environmentally modulated. elife 6
9. Saraiva LR, Ahuja G, Ivandic I, Syed AS, Marioni JC, Korsching SI, Logan DW (2015) Molecular and neuronal homology between the olfactory systems of zebrafish and mouse. Sci Rep 5:11487
10. Saraiva LR, Ibarra-Soria X, Khan M, Omura M, Scialdone A, Mombaerts P, Marioni JC, Logan DW (2015) Hierarchical deconstruction of mouse olfactory sensory neurons: from whole mucosa to single-cell RNA-seq. Sci Rep 5: 18178
11. Horowitz LF, Saraiva LR, Kuang D, Yoon KH, Buck LB (2014) Olfactory receptor patterning in a higher primate. J Neurosci 34:12241–12252

12. Ibarra-Soria X, Levitin MO, Saraiva LR, Logan DW (2014) The olfactory transcriptomes of mice. PLoS Genet 10:e1004593
13. Asp M, Bergenstrahle J, Lundeberg J (2020) Spatially resolved transcriptomes-next generation tools for tissue exploration. Bioessays 42 (10):e1900221
14. Junker JP, Noel ES, Guryev V, Peterson KA, Shah G, Huisken J, McMahon AP, Berezikov E, Bakkers J, van Oudenaarden A (2014) Genome-wide RNA Tomography in the zebrafish embryo. Cell 159:662–675
15. Ruiz Tejada Segura ML, Abou Moussa E, Garabello E, Nakahara TS, Makhlouf M, Mathew LS, Wang L, Valle F, Huang SSY, Mainland JD et al (2022) A 3D transcriptomics atlas of the mouse nose sheds light on the anatomical logic of smell. Cell Rep 38:110547

Chapter 3

Optical Activation of Photoswitchable TRPC Ligands in the Mammalian Olfactory System Using Laser Scanning Confocal Microscopy

Navin K. Ojha, Frank Zufall, and Trese Leinders-Zufall

Abstract

The transient receptor potential canonical (TRPC) ion channels play important biological roles, but their activation mechanisms are incompletely understood. Here, we describe recent methodological advances using small molecular probes designed for photopharmacology of TRPC channels by focusing on results obtained from the mouse olfactory system. These studies developed and used photoswitchable diacylglycerol (DAG) analogs for ultrarapid activation of native TRPC2 channels in vomeronasal sensory neurons and type B cells of the main olfactory epithelium. Further studies investigated the role of TRPC5 channels in prolactin regulation of dopamine neurons in the arcuate nucleus of the hypothalamus. Here, the first photoswitchable TRPC5 modulator, BTDAzo, was developed and shown to control endogenous TRPC5-based neuronal Ca^{2+} responses in mouse brain slices. Thus, photoswitchable reagents are rapidly gaining widespread recognition for investigating various types of TRPC channels including TRPC2, TRPC3, TRPC5, and TRPC6, enabling to gain new insights into the gating mechanisms and functions of these channels.

Key words TRP channel, Photopharmacology, PhoDAG, BTDAzo, Biosensor, Prolactin, Olfaction, Vomeronasal, Hypothalamus, Lipid signaling

1 Introduction

Transient receptor potential (TRP) channels of the TRPC (canonical) subfamily play important roles in the mammalian olfactory system. They were first discovered in peripheral sensory neurons of the olfactory system, but more recently, efforts have been made to characterize TRPC channel function also in higher centers of the olfactory pathway such as specific regions of the hypothalamus.

The first molecularly defined TRP channel found in the mouse olfactory system was TRPC2, identified more than two decades ago in the vomeronasal sensory neurons (VSNs) of the accessory olfactory system (also known as vomeronasal system) (Fig. 1)

Bradley J. Goldstein and Hiroaki Matsunami (eds.), *The Olfactory System*, Methods in Molecular Biology, vol. 2710, https://doi.org/10.1007/978-1-0716-3425-7_3,

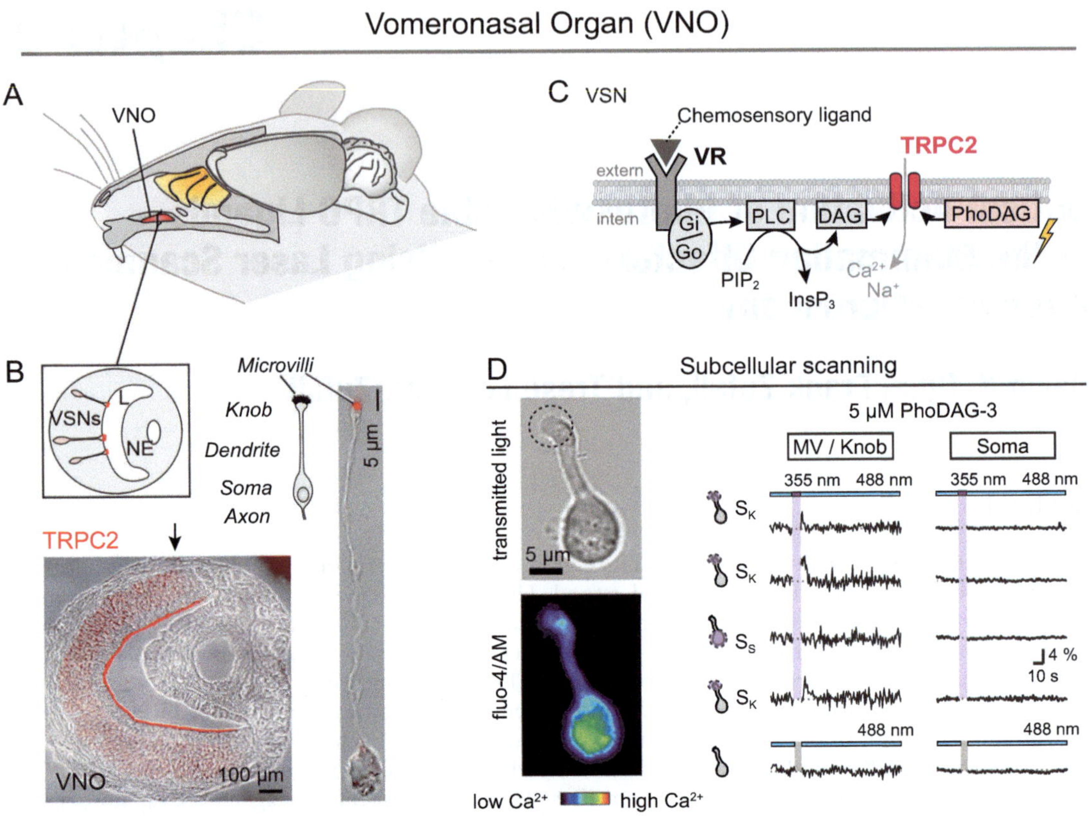

Fig. 1 (**a**) Sagittal view of a mouse head indicating the location of the VNO (*red*). (**b**) Coronal section through the VNO showing the crescent-shaped VNO sensory epithelium containing single VSNs. The immunohistochemical fluorescence images indicate that TRPC2 (*red*) is located at the luminal surface of the sensory epithelium and mainly restricted to the microvilli. Fluorescence images reproduced from Proc. Natl. Acad. Sci. USA with permission (Copyright, 1999, National Academy of Sciences, USA) [2]. (**c**) Model of chemoelectrical signal transduction in VSNs. Central in this pathway is the Ca^{2+} permeable TRPC2 channel. The only known activator of TRPC2 is diacylglycerol (DAG), most likely produced by phospholipase C (PLC) that in turn is stimulated by either the Gi-coupled vomeronasal receptor (VR) of type 1 or the Go-coupled VR of type 2. (**d**) Combined optical photoswitching and Ca^{2+} imaging of a dissociated VSN loaded with the photoswitchable ligand PhoDAG-3 (5 μM) and the Ca^{2+} indicator fluo-4/AM (9 μM). Subcellular structures of a dissociated VSN are shown in the transmitted light and confocal fluorescence images (pseudocolor scale; acquired at rest). The dashed circle indicates the VSN dendritic ending containing the microvilli and dendritic knob. Spatially localized photoswitching (355 nm, magenta) of PhoDAG-3 at the dendritic knob and microvilli (SK) produced Ca^{2+} transients at the microvilli/knob region (MV/Knob) but not at the soma. Localized photoswitching at the soma (SS) produced no Ca^{2+} responses at all. (Reproduced from Elsevier with permission [9])

[1–3]. Ever since, TRPC2 has played a central role in the signal transduction machinery of the VSNs and in identifying VNO-based behavioral responses and even the central circuits underlying VNO-mediated social behaviors (for a review, see [4]). After 20 years of intense research, the only second messenger molecule that has been shown to activate TRPC2 or TRPC2-based cellular responses is the membrane lipid diacylglycerol (DAG) produced by the enzyme phospholipase C [5, 6]. By contrast, genetic deletion of inositol 1,4,5-trisphosphate ($InsP_3$) signaling had no obvious effect on primary signal transduction in VSNs [7]. The TRPC2 channels are permeable for Ca^{2+}, which does not activate the channel but, in combination with calmodulin (CaM), inhibits TRPC2 activity to mediate Ca^{2+}-CaM dependent negative feedback regulation – required for sensory adaptation and plasticity of the VSNs [6]. Despite these abundant results, the activation of TRPC2 by DAG was not fully accepted. We therefore set out to develop optical methods that would provide precise spatiotemporal control over the activation and deactivation of TRPC2-mediated currents and Ca^{2+} responses within their native cellular environment. This goal was recently achieved when we used a unique family of light-sensitive, photoswitchable diacylglycerols, known as PhoDAGs [8, 9]. The results revealed that brief photoactivation of two distinct PhoDAG analogs for less than 30 ms is sufficient to activate native TRPC2 channels and produce a concomitant Ca^{2+} rise in VSNs [9, 10]. Furthermore, the activation of TRPC2-mediated currents could be reversed and switched off by photoswitching the PhoDAG back into its inactive form, and this activation/deactivation could be repeated over multiple cycles [9]. Together, these results provided definitive evidence that TRPC2 is a diacylglycerol-sensitive ion channel.

Although TRPC2 was initially thought to be expressed selectively in VSNs, more recent work has identified in the mouse main olfactory epithelium (MOE) two previously unrecognized types of sensory neurons that also express TRPC2, together with the cyclic nucleotide-gated channel subunit CNGA2 (Fig. 2) [11, 12]. These cells were termed type A and type B cells. We undertook intense efforts to identify the signaling mechanisms and biological functions of the type B cells [13, 14]. During the course of these studies, we also investigated whether TRPC2 is a functional channel in both cell types by performing DAG photoswitching experiments [9, 10]. These results clearly revealed that both type A and type B cells exhibit DAG-evoked cellular responses, whereas classical olfactory sensory neurons (OSNs) of the MOE do not [9]. TRPC2 knockout studies showed that this channel is required for the detection of low environmental oxygen in the type B cells and that these cells mediate danger perception and stress responses through TRPC2 signaling [13, 14]. Thus, DAG-sensitive TRPC2 channels are now known to play important roles in both the VNO and the MOE.

We also undertook efforts to identify the roles of additional TRPC channel functions in higher centers of the olfactory system, in combination with novel TRPC channel photoswitching methodology (Fig. 3) [15, 16]. Specifically, we focused on a set of dopamine neurons in the arcuate nucleus (ARC) of the hypothalamus, which receive olfactory sensory input and which play a crucial

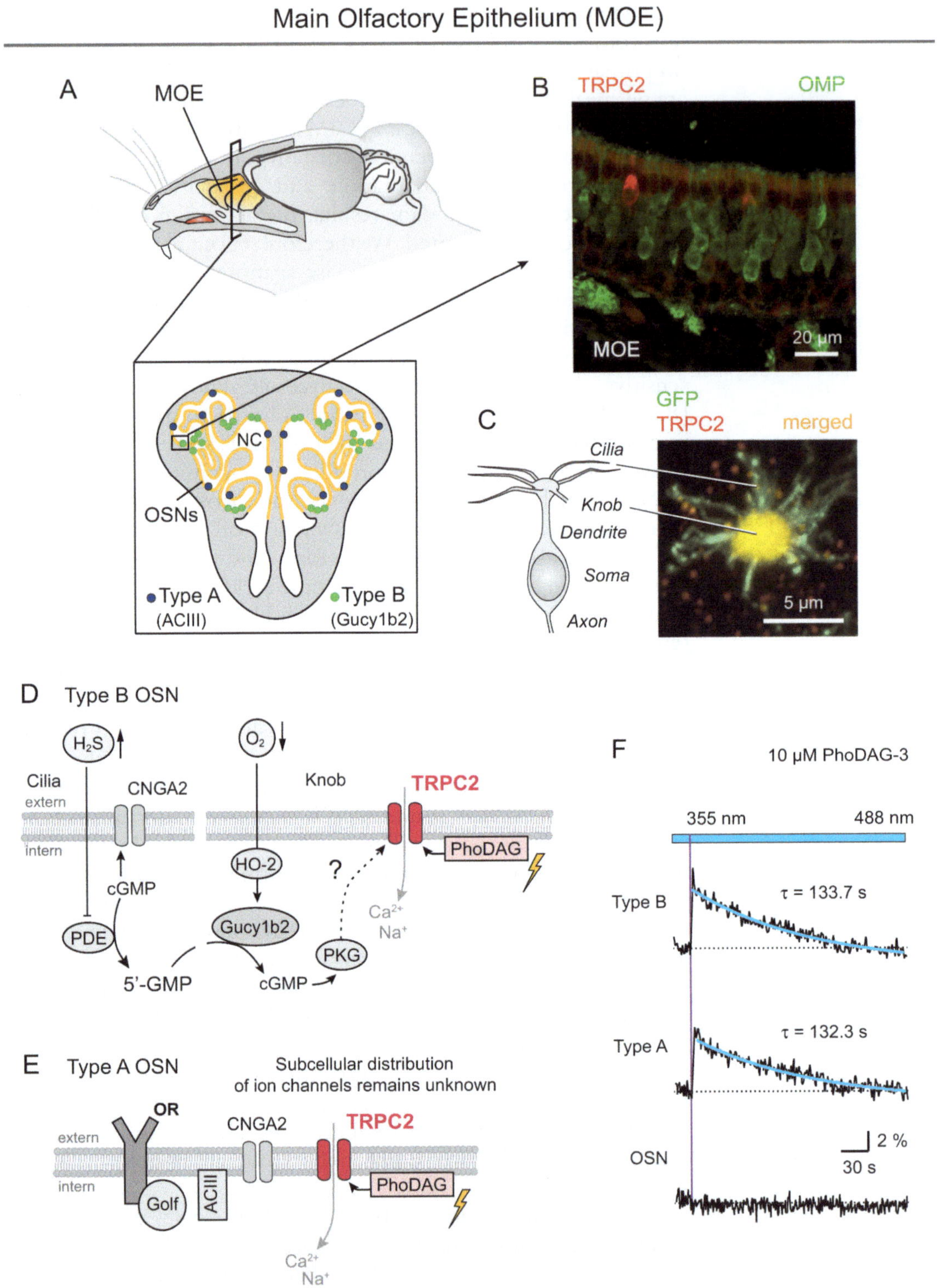

Fig. 2 (**a**) Sagittal view of a mouse head indicating the location of the MOE (*yellow*) and the scheme of a coronal section through the nasal cavity containing the MOE tissue. The location of the two types of TRPC2-expressing OSNs co-expressing either adenylyl cyclase III (ACIII) or the soluble guanylyl cyclase type 1b2 (Gucy1b2) is indicated in blue and green dots, respectively. (**b**) Immunohistochemical fluorescence indicating

role in the regulation of prolactin homeostasis of the body [15]. We found that the ion channel TRPC5 is a major determinant of hypothalamic prolactin regulation and defines the functional properties of the dopaminergic ARC neurons [15]. TRPC5 is of special interest because of its potential importance in metabolic medicine (see [16]). The activation mechanism of TRPC5 is currently not fully understood, but there is evidence that TRPC5 could also be a DAG-sensitive ion channel [17]. In the context of these and other studies, the first photoswitchable TRPC5 modulator, BTDAzo, was recently developed and shown to control endogenous TRPC5-based neuronal Ca^{2+} responses in mouse hypothalamic brain slices (Fig. 3) [16]. Thus multiple types of TRPC channels are expressed within the olfactory system where they perform important biological functions, and small molecular probes designed for photopharmacology and opto-chemogenetics are rapidly becoming important tools to investigate these functions.

We note that, in addition to members of the TRPC channel subfamily, there is now also evidence for emerging roles of TRPM (melastatin) channels such as TRPM4 and TRPM5 in the mammalian olfactory system (e.g., see [18, 19]). As these are Ca^{2+}-activated monovalent cation channels, most likely dependent on $InsP_3$-mediated signaling mechanisms, both photoreleasable Ca^{2+} or $InsP_3$ (e.g., see [7]) can be used to investigate the functions of these channels in the olfactory system with high spatial and temporal resolution.

Here, we will briefly summarize the methods that have enabled the use of photoswitchable reagents as powerful tools for high-precision biological control of TRPC channels in three different regions of the mammalian olfactory system: the VNO, the MOE, and the hypothalamus. Additional information on these methods can be found in the original reports [9, 10, 16].

Fig. 2 (continued) the presence of TRPC2 (*red*)-expressing OSNs within the olfactory marker protein (OMP, green) expressing mature OSNs (merged (*yellow*): coexpression of TRPC2 and OMP). Reproduced from Cell Press with permission [11]. (**c**) Confocal en face images of a type B OSN from a Gucy1b2-GFP mouse in a whole-mount preparation showing GFP (*green*) and Trpc2 immunoreactivity (*red*) which was confined to the dendritic knob (*yellow*). Reproduced from Cell Press with permission [14]. (**d** and **e**) Model of chemoelectrical signal transduction in type B (**d**) and type A (**e**) OSNs. Type B OSNs use an alternative signaling logic that utilizes CNGA2 and TRPC2 channels mediated detection within the same chemosensory neuron. This strategy serves to facilitate the integration and coincidence detection of at least two poisonous environmental chemical conditions, namely, the increase in H_2S or the decrease in O_2. In response to these life-threatening chemicals, the hypothalamus-pituitary-adrenal (HPA) axis is activated, an effective stress mechanism to increase survival chances of the individual. In type A OSNs, only key signaling molecules have been identified: olfactory receptors (OR), G-protein (Golf), adenylyl cyclase III (ACIII), the cyclic nucleotide-gated type A2 (CNGA2), and TRPC2 channels. (F) Combined optical photoswitching and Ca^{2+} imaging of a dissociated type B and type A OSN loaded with the photoswitchable ligand PhoDAG-3 (10 μM) and the Ca^{2+} indicator fluo-4/AM (9 μM). Photostimulation (355 nm, thin magenta line) of PhoDAG-3 caused Ca^{2+} transients in both type B and A OSNs. No responses occurred in classical OSNs. (Reproduced from Elsevier with permission [9])

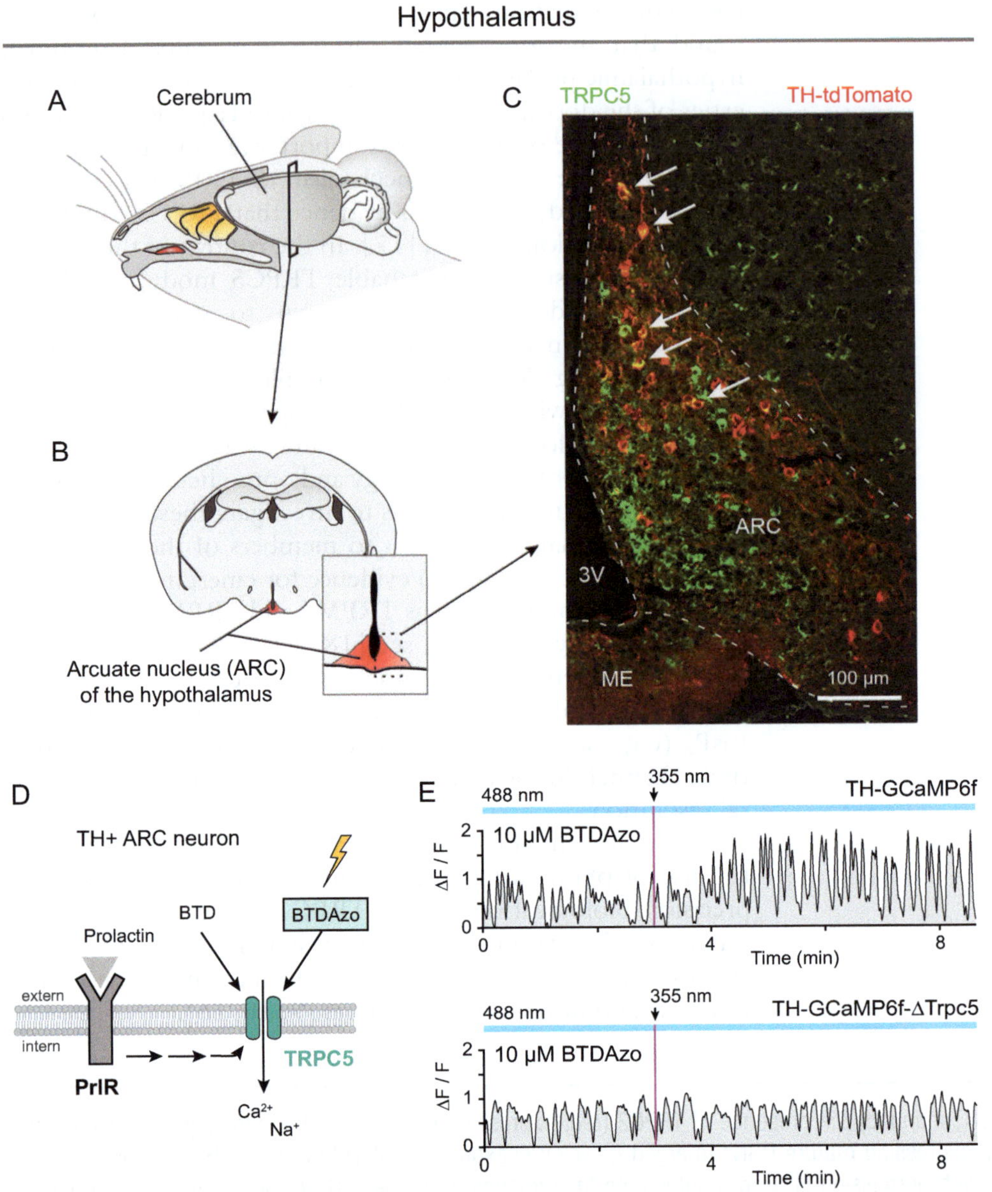

Fig. 3 (**a** and **b**) Sagittal view of a mouse head (**a**) indicating the location of the coronal section containing the arcuate nucleus (*red*) of the hypothalamus (**b**). (**c**) Immunohistochemical confocal image of one side of the hypothalamic arcuate nucleus (ARC) containing TRPC5 (*green*) expression in dopaminergic neurons (*red*) of Th-tdTomato mice (TH-cre x Rosa26-tdTomato, TH, tyrosine hydroxylase). White arrows indicate the TH+ TRPC5+ neurons (*yellow*). (**d**) Model of electrical signal transduction in TH+ TRPC5+ ARC neurons. Both prolactin-evoked responses and the responses to the TRPC5 agonist BTD in these neurons require TRPC5 [15, 16]. (**e**) Combined optical photoswitching and Ca^{2+} imaging in TH+ ARC neurons from TH-GCaMP6f mice which genetically express the Ca^{2+} indicator GCaMP6f and which were loaded with the photoswitchable agonist BTDAzo (10 μM). Photostimulation (355 nm, thin magenta line) caused an increase in amplitude and the frequency of the spontaneous Ca^{2+} transients in these neurons of TH-GCaMP6f mice in contrast to the TRPC5-deficient mouse line (TH-GCaMP6f-ΔTrpc5). (Reproduced from Wiley-VCH with permission [16])

2 Materials

2.1 Preparation of Physiological Solutions

Use commercially available analytical grade chemical reagents and ultrapure water (>18.2 MΩ cm resistivity at 25 °C, low ppt in divalent cations) for the preparation of all physiological solutions. Various ultrapure water systems are available which filter pretreated water (reverse osmosis or demineralized water) to produce water with <5 ppb total organic carbon (TOC).

Prepare extracellular solution 1 (S1) in ultrapure water according to the table below (Table 1). The osmolarity of the solution will be 300 mOsm/kg if all chemicals were weighed correctly. Filter the solution using a 0.2 μm membrane filter to eliminate dust particles and possible microbial contaminants. The pH of the solution will be ~7.3 when aerated with carbogen (95% O_2 / 5% CO_2) for ~10 min. Store the solution at 4 °C. Bring the solution to room temperature before its use.

2.2 Preparation of Photoswitchable Ligands

Several photoswitchable reagents are now available that have been shown to activate TRPC2, TRPC3, TRPC5, or TRPC6 channels, and these are summarized in Fig. 4 (adapted and modified from [10]). The general steps of dissolving these chemicals are described in the following section and depicted in Fig. 5a.

1. Dissolve the photoswitchable ligand in anhydrous DMSO (*see* **Notes 1**) as indicated (*see* **Notes 2**):
   (a) 100 mM PhoDAG-1 stock solution: 5 mg PhoDAG-1 (1-stearoyl-2-[(E)-4-(4-((4-butylphenyl)diazenyl)phenyl)butanoyl]-sn-glycerol; MW = 664.970 Da; Fig. 4; [9, 20]), also known as 18:0-PhoDAG (Sigma/Aldrich or CD-Bioparticles) in 75.19 μl anhydrous DMSO (dimethyl sulfoxide).

Table 1
Extracellular solution (S1)

Reagents		Amount (mmol)
NaCl	Sodium chloride	120
$NaHCO_3$	Sodium hydrogen carbonate	25
KCl	Potassium chloride	5
$C_6H_{15}NO_5S$	BES (2-hydroxyethyl)-2 aminoethanesulfonic acid	5
$MgSO_4$	Magnesium sulfate	1
$CaCl_2$	Calcium chloride	1
$C_6H_{12}O_6$	D(+)-Glucose	10

Mix all reagents in 1 l ultrapure water

Photoswitchable Ligands of TRPC Ion Channels

	channel closed 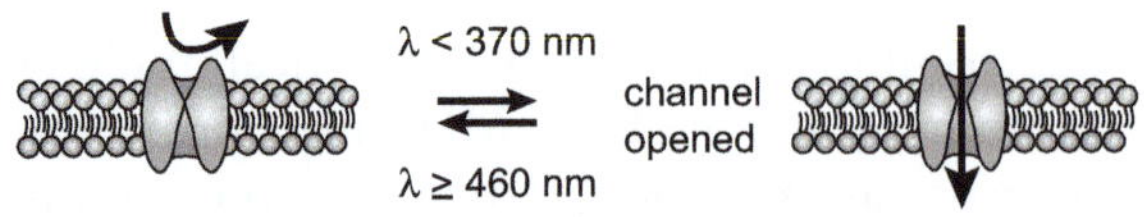 channel opened		Ion channel	Effective concentration [Reference]
PhoDAG-3	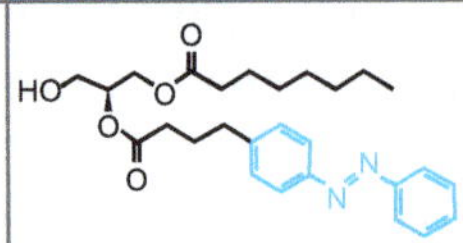	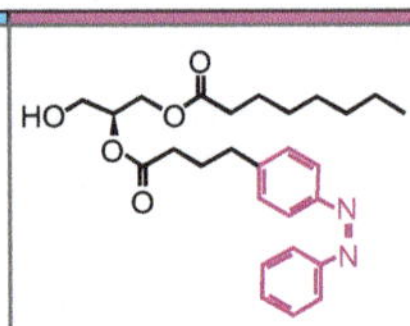	**mTRPC2**	5, 10, 50 µM [9]
PhoDAG-1 = 18:0-PhoDAG	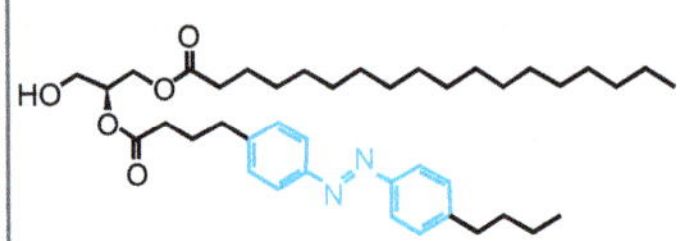	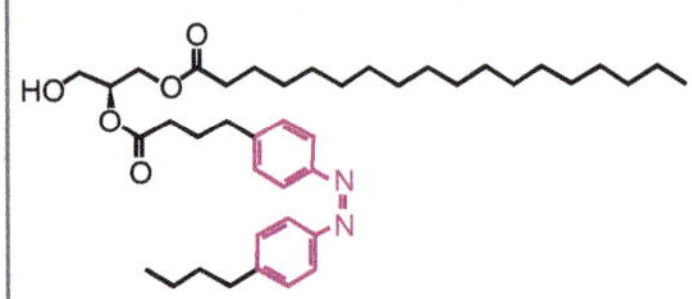	**mTRPC2**	10 µM [9]
			hTRPC3	400 µM [27]
			hTRPC6	100 µM [9]
OptoDArG	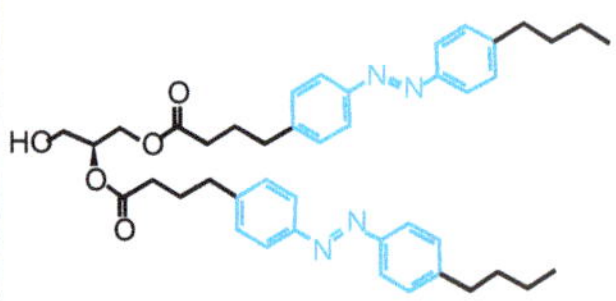	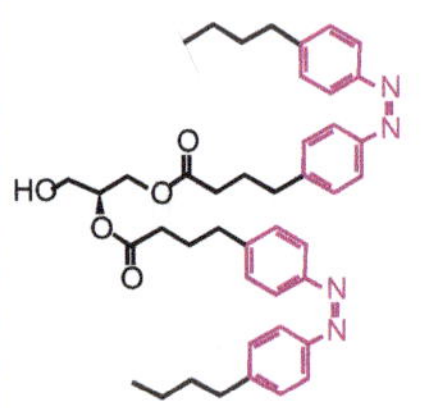	**mTRPC2**	30 µM [10]
			hTRPC3	30 µM [27]
			hTRPC6	30 µM [10]
BTDAzo	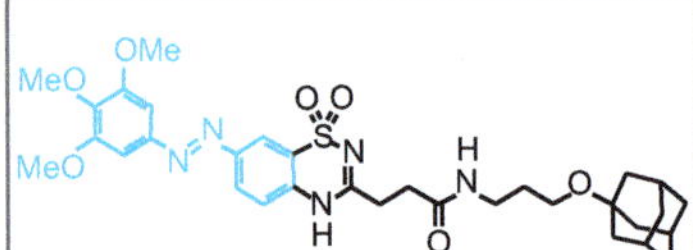	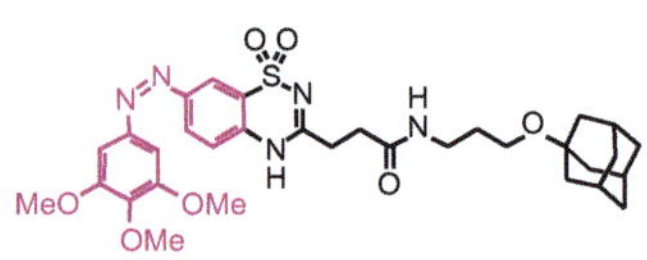	**mTRPC5**	10 µM [16]
			hTRPC5	

Fig. 4 Chemical structures of known photoswitchable ligands for TRPC ion channels. The photoswitchable diacylglycerols (PhoDAG-3, PhoDAG-1 with its new commercial name 18:0-PhoDAG, and OptoDArG) as well as the TRPC5 agonist (BTDAzo) change their configuration in response to UV-A ($\lambda < 370$ nm) and blue ($\lambda \geq 460$ nm) illumination, respectively. The diacylglycerol (DAG) analogs have been shown to activate mouse TRPC2, human TRPC3, and human TRPC6 channels

(b) 100 mM OptoDArG stock solution: 5 mg OptoDArG (3-Hydroxypropane-1,2-diyl-bis(4-(4-((E)-(4-butylphenyl)diazenyl)phenyl)butanoate; MW = 704.39 Da; Fig. 4; [10, 20]) in 70.98 µl anhydrous DMSO.

(c) 20 mM stock of BTDAzo: 3.2 mg BTDAzo (MW = 639.8 Da; Fig. 4; [16]) in 250 µl anhydrous DMSO.

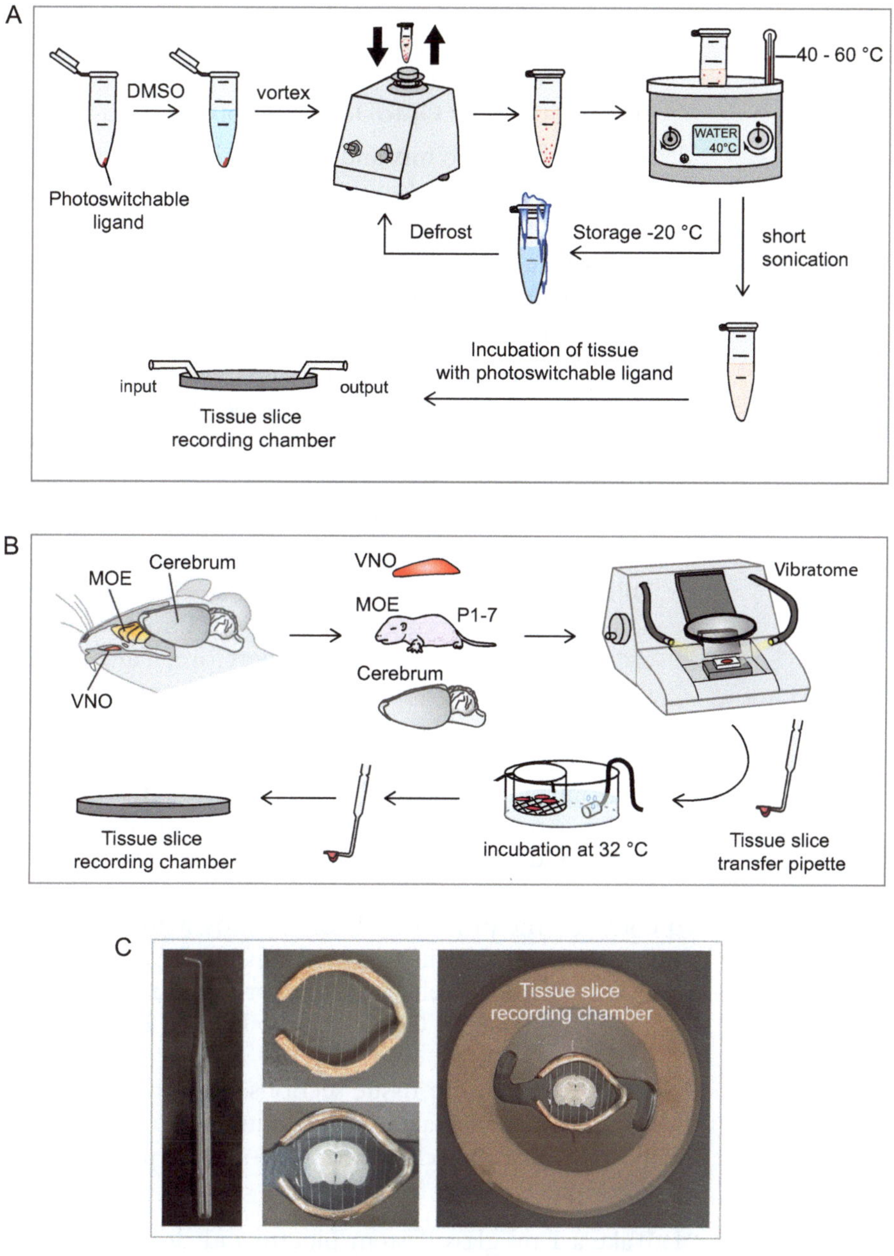

Fig. 5 (**a**) Pictogram of the steps for the solubilization of photoswitchable ligands (see Subheading 2.2 for details). (**b**) Pictogram of the steps for producing tissue slices and transferring them from the vibratome to the incubation chamber and then to the recording chamber (see Subheadings 2.4 and 3). (**c**) Photographs of the tissue slice transfer pipette (left), the tissue slice holder (harp), which is made of a parallel array of nylon threads strung on an oval shaped platinum/silver frame without (middle upper) or with a mouse coronal brain slice (middle lower), and the top view of a laminar flow recording chamber containing a mouse coronal brain section secured by the harp to avoid movement caused by the speed of the solution flow through the chamber (right). Note that the harp is shaped so that the flow of the solution is not hindered by the wire, as it has an opening at the inlet and a bridge at the outlet

2. Warm the solution to a temperature between 40 and 60 °C for 5 to 10 min to help dissolve the photoswitchable ligands. Optimal temperatures are ~40 °C for PhoDAG-1, between 40 and 60 °C for OptoDArG and 60 °C for BTDAzo.
3. Sonicate briefly to mix and dissolve the photoswitchable ligand completely. Avoid long sonication. If the photoswitchable ligand is not completely dissolved, repeat step 2.
4. Aliquot the photoswitchable ligand stock solution in portions of 10–100 μl, and store them in a desiccator at −20 °C for long-term use (1–6 months).
5. To make the working solution, take out a frozen stock aliquot, and let it equilibrate to room temperature in a desiccator. The anhydrous DMSO will otherwise attract water (condensation) which will alter the concentration.
6. Repeat steps 2 and 3 to ensure the photoswitchable ligand is completely dissolved.
7. Dilute the photoswitchable ligand stock solution using S1 to achieve a final working concentration. Photoswitchable ligands are sparingly soluble in water. Therefore, if any of them precipitate from the S1 solution, warm it up to ~40 °C, and then sonicate briefly. The percentage of DMSO in the final working solution should not be greater than 0.1% (vol/vol). The working solution of photoswitchable ligands can also be stored at −20 °C. Bring the solution to room temperature before its use. Warm and sonicate again if needed.

2.3 Preparation of Ca^{2+}-Indicator Dye Solution

To combine the photoswitchable ligands with Ca^{2+} imaging on a confocal microscope, fluo-4/AM can be used as a Ca^{2+} indicator dye (*see* **Notes 1**) if cells are not expressing a genetically encoded Ca^{2+} indicator such as GCaMP6f [9, 10, 16, 21, 22].

2.4 Preparation of Tissue Slice Transfer Pipette

For the transfer of live tissue sections from the slicing chamber of the vibratome to an aerated S1 solution-containing beaker and finally to a recording chamber, an L-shaped pipette is made from a Pasteur pipette (Fig. 5b, c).

1. Take a 1 ml glass Pasteur pipette and close the opening of the Pasteur pipette tip by holding it over the flame of a gas burner.
2. Heat the glass Pasteur pipette slowly at about 1–1.5 cm from the tip of the narrow area.
3. Bend the heated glass section of the Pasteur pipette into an L-shaped hook, and allow it to cool.

3 Methods

Detailed descriptions of the procedures for obtaining (I) mouse chemosensory neurons expressing TRPC2 channels from (a) the vomeronasal organ (VNO) or (b) the main olfactory epithelium (MOE), and (II) dopaminergic neurons from neuroendocrine cells in the mouse hypothalamus expressing TRPC5 channels (Figs. 1, 2, 3, and 5b, c) have been published previously [10, 15, 16, 23]. Before beginning any animal experimental procedure, you should apply for approval and strictly follow the guidelines established by the animal welfare committee of your institution.

3.1 Optical Activation of Photoswitchable TRPC Ligands Using Laser Scanning Confocal Microscopy

1. The recording setup (*see* **Notes 3** and **4**): A critical advantage of laser scanning technology is that it enables precise spatial and temporal control over the photoswitch. For example, spatially localized photoswitching can be obtained within small subcellular compartments such as cilia, microvilli, and dendritic endings of olfactory neurons [9]. Laser scanning illumination can also be used to perform large-scale mapping of cellular activity across a population of cells in a tissue slice or an entire organ [9, 10, 16].

   For combined acquisition of calcium signals and stimulation (photoswitching) of a light-sensitive ligand in tissue slices or cells, an upright scanning confocal microscope has to be equipped with an Argon laser (488 nm) for excitation of fluo4/AM or GCaMP6f and a UV 355 nm laser for photoswitching the TRPC ligands (Fig. 1d, 2f, 3e, 6a). Additional modification to the confocal microscope includes a shutter to protect the PMT against damaging high-intensity laser light necessary for photoswitching the ligands (Fig. 6a). Depending on the confocal microscope and the light pathway, two scanning mirrors and at least two different dichroic beamsplitters are required (Fig. 6a). We use an upright scanning confocal microscope (Zeiss LSM 880 INDIMO) with individualized modifications performed by Zeiss which include the use of any type of laser wavelength for recording or stimulating/photoswitching.

2. Cells/slices loaded with a calcium indicator or expressing a genetic indicator such as GCaMP6f are placed in a laminar flow recording chamber (Fig. 5c) and continuously perfused with extracellular S1 solution (aerated with 95% O_2 / 5% CO_2) at an appropriate flow rate (e.g., 100 μl/s) to ensure the health of the cells. Tissue slices, like a mouse coronal brain section, are secured by a tissue slice holder (harp) to avoid movement caused by the speed of the solution flow through the chamber (Fig. 5c). Control the flow of the bath perfusion solution, e.g., with a pump or gravity feed. The solution speed in a gravity feed system should be strictly controlled using a combination

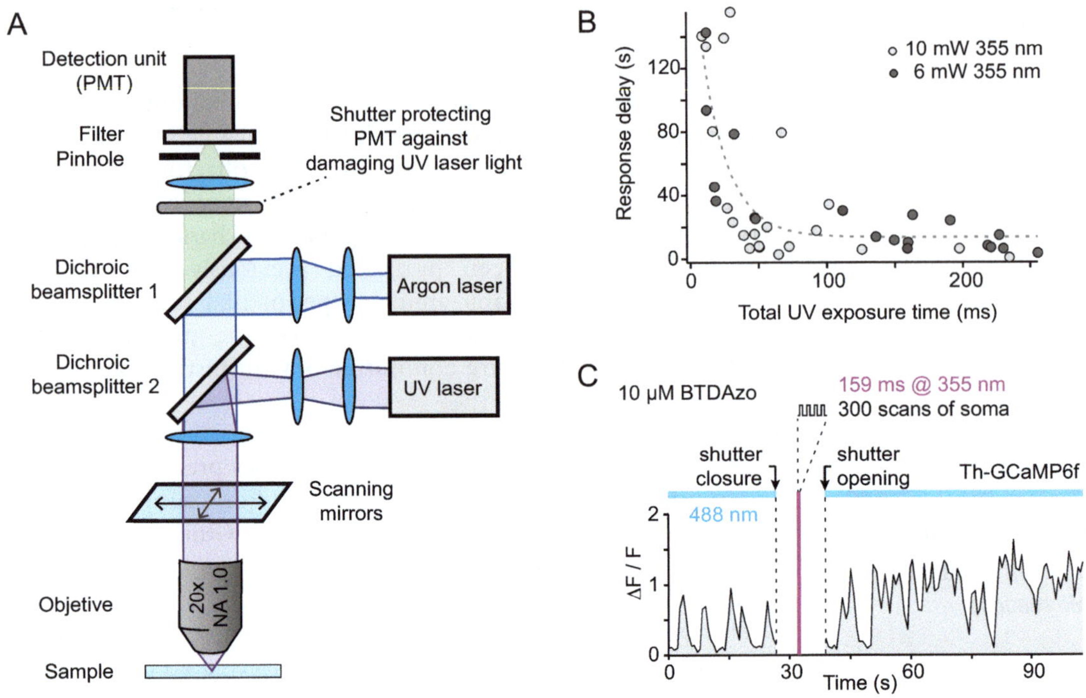

Fig. 6 (**a**) Schematic of the light path for an upright confocal laser scanning microscope that includes modifications to allow the combined use of an UV laser (355 nm) for photomanipulation and an argon laser (488 nm) for excitation of Ca^{2+} indicators such as fluo-4 or GCaMP6f without damaging the sensitive photomultiplier tubes (PMT); see also **Notes 7**. (**b**) The response delay vs. UV exposure time plot indicates the minimum UV light exposure required to induce the shortest response time to photocontrol BTDAzo-induced Ca^{2+} responses in TH+ neurons (see Fig. 3). Optimal UV exposure time in the brain slices was >120 ms to obtain the fastest photocontrol ranging between 0.7 and 27.5 s. (**c**) Example of an optimized protocol to photoswitch BTDAzo to activate TRPC5-dependent Ca^{2+} increase in TH+ neurons. UV stimulation (6 mW 355 nm) consisted of 300 individual scans of the cell soma with a pixel dwell time of 0.82 μs which resulted in a total UV exposure time of 159 ms. (**b** and **c**). (Reproduced from Wiley-VCH with permission [16])

of solution volume (container) and gravity flow controllers. Keep track of the perfusion solution volume to maintain relatively equal pressure on the tubing lines. Check once using food color in the perfusion system how the solution will spread and exchange in the recording chamber and under the 20 × 1.0 NA Plan-Apochromat water immersion objective.

3. Visualize the cells within a scanning field (x, y) of 512 × 512 pixels and a depth (z, optical section thickness) of ~10–20 μm. The thickness of the optical section should not be too thin since this would prevent sufficient illumination of the photoswitchable ligands in the membrane and perhaps damage cells of interest with too much laser power.

4. Adjust the pixel dwell time of the laser to a total image scanning field (x, y) of 512 × 512 pixels to ~1 s.

5. Draw regions of interests (ROIs) via the acquisition software tool (Zen, Zeiss), and measure the basic activity of the cells, and ensure there is no drift in the calcium imaging recording using the Argon laser (488 nm) for 4 min. The acquisition software (Zen, Zeiss) will capture the emission fluorescence (510–560 nm). All scanning head settings need to be kept constant during the whole experiment to ensure comparison of the image data. At 488 nm wavelength, preloaded photoswitchable ligands are mainly in the inactive form.
6. Add and incubate the cells/tissue slice with the photoswitchable ligand. The time required for loading photoswitchable ligands into living cells can vary greatly and depends on the particular cell type and the chemical structure of a given ligand. In our experience, it takes between 20 and 30 min at room temperature in the dark. During a stable physiological recording, it is possible to measure the response before, during loading and after sufficient loading to determine the optimal time for loading a particular opto-ligand.
7. Scan preselected regions of interests (ROIs) via the acquisition software tool (Zeiss Zen, "Bleaching") to photoswitch the opto-ligand to its active form using UV light of 355 nm. To prevent damage to the highly sensitive gallium-arsenide-phosphide (GaAsP) detectors, a preinstalled shutter should be activated which will block UV light reaching the detector (Fig. 6d). The collection of the calcium indicator fluorescence is halted during photoswitching of the opto-ligands but resumes at the end of the UV stimulation.
8. Optimize the activation of the photoswitchable ligands by performing UV stimulation with different intensities (coherent UV laser: 1–60 mW) and UV exposure times (*see* **Notes 4, 5** and **6**) to produce a calcium fluorescence response delay (see point 9) vs. total UV exposure time plot. In our experiments (Fig. 6b, c), UV exposure consisted of pulsed laser scanning of the ROI with either (i) 300 individual scans of the cell soma having a pixel dwell time of 0.82 μs or 1.02 μs or (ii) 100 individual scans of the cell soma having a pixel dwell time of 2.05 μs to obtain a total UV exposure time >120 ms and the fastest response of around 11 s.

   An example for calculating total UV exposure time: for a single neuron with a size of approximately 154 μm^2, a UV stimulation could consist of 10 individual scans of this ROI (647 pixels with a pixel size of 0.238 μm^2). Given a laser dwell time of 2.05 μs/pixel, the duration of UV exposure (= number of scans x area (pixels) x dwell time/pixel) will thus be 13.3 ms.
9. Analyze Ca^{2+} images using a combination of the acquisition software (Zeiss Zen), ImageJ (NIH), and Igor Pro (WaveMetrics) software. The onset time of Ca^{2+} signal is defined as

the difference between the time point at which 488 nm excitation started after UV exposure and the time at which Ca^{2+} fluorescence exceeded twice the standard deviation of the mean of the baseline noise. To quantify the changes in the dynamics of Ca^{2+} responses in intrinsically active neurons (oscillating dopaminergic neurons; Fig. 3e) [16], the area under the curve (AUC) can be calculated as a measure for the increase in intracellular Ca^{2+}. A control AUC is taken at the beginning of a recording for 3 min. The AUC after activating a photoswitchable ligand is then calculated from the last 3 min of the total 9 min recording (basic activity and after UV stimulation). The Ca^{2+} fluorescence response delay is the subtraction of the time at the end of the UV exposure from the onset time of the Ca^{2+} signal change (*see* **Note 8**).

10. Besides using laser scanning illumination, we have also described step-by-step methods for using fiber-coupled light-emitting diodes (LEDs) or a monochromator for photoswitching of TRPC channel ligands [10].

4 Notes

1. DMSO is known to affect the integrity of the cell membrane and thus could alter the physiological response under investigation [24, 25]. Therefore, the concentration of the stock solution of the photoswitchable ligand should be carefully considered because of its influence on the solution containing the final DMSO concentration that is delivered to the cells. A DMSO concentration of $\leq$0.1% should be sufficient to keep the compound in solution and not harm most cells. Cell lines appear to be less susceptible to DMSO damage compared with native cells. Control experiments should be performed with solutions containing the final DMSO concentration without the photoswitchable ligand.
2. The production of photoswitchable ligands does not have to occur in the dark. Exposure to darkness converts these molecules back to their inactive form [8, 9].
3. Prior to photoswitching, UV laser light should be optimally focused in 18-mm-thick tissue sections by loading them with a nuclear stain, such as Hoechst 33342 (1:10000). The semiautomatic correction tool of the Zen software (Zeiss) facilitates this calibration.
4. The UV laser power has to be adjusted depending on the photoswitchable ligand used and the final concentration introduced into the cells. PhoDAG-1 and PhoDAG-3 could be switched to the active cis-form with a UV laser power of 10 mW. However, for OptoDArG, 30 mW of laser power was required to achieve a similar Ca^{2+} response [10].

5. Confirm that the cellular responses are not affected by the UV light or other laser wavelengths (phototoxicity) [26, 27]. The uploaded amount of the photoswitchable ligands needs to be optimized in relation to the laser light intensity. Another solution to reduce phototoxicity is to shorten the illumination time by changing the exposure time or the pixel dwell time. However, this should be weighed in relation to the cellular response to be measured.
6. The active form of the photoswitchable ligand stimulated by UV light may not switch back to the inactive form. In this case, cells could be damaged by a sustained inward current and accumulation of intracellular Ca^{2+}. Complete darkness or an increase in the intensity of the laser light with a $\geq$ 450 nm wavelength may help to switch the photoswitchable ligand back to its inactive form.
7. Low laser intensity of 488 nm is required for Ca^{2+} imaging. This could limit the formation of the inactive form of the photoswitchable ligands and keep some of the molecules in their active form. One solution would be to have a third laser line available that does not excite the calcium indicator dye but helps to convert the photoswitchable ligand to the inactive form. This third laser could use the same light path as the UV laser (Fig. 6a).
8. Rule out off-target effects in experiments with native cells by using knockout mice. We have used TRPC2 knockout mice as controls for photoswitching experiments in VSNs and found no current activation under these conditions, thus ruling out any off-target effects [9]. Similarly, we performed experiments with TRPC5-deficient mice to confirm the targeting of the photoswitchable ligand BTDAzo in hypothalamic neuroendocrine cells [16].

Acknowledgments

This work was supported by Deutsche Forschungsgemeinschaft (DFG) Grants Sonderforschungsbereich-Transregio TRR 152 and SFB 894 (to F.Z. and T.L.-Z.), DFG Instrumentation Grant INST 256/427-1 FUGB (to T.L.-Z.), and the Volkswagen Foundation (to T.L.-Z.). We thank the groups of Dirk Trauner, Thomas Gudermann, Michael Schaefer and Oliver Thorn-Seshold for their contributions to the work described here.

References

1. Leypold BG, Yu CR, Leinders-Zufall T, Kim MM, Zufall F, Axel R (2002) Altered sexual and social behaviors in trp2 mutant mice. Proc Natl Acad Sci U S A 99:6376–6381
2. Liman ER, Corey DP, Dulac C (1999) TRP2: a candidate transduction channel for mammalian pheromone sensory signaling. Proc Natl Acad Sci U S A 96:5791–5796
3. Stowers L, Holy TE, Meister M, Dulac C, Koentges G (2002) Loss of sex discrimination and male-male aggression in mice deficient for TRP2. Science 295:1493–1500
4. Chamero P, Leinders-Zufall T, Zufall F (2012) From genes to social communication: molecular sensing by the vomeronasal organ. Trends Neurosci 35:597–606
5. Lucas P, Ukhanov K, Leinders-Zufall T, Zufall F (2003) A diacylglycerol-gated cation channel in vomeronasal neuron dendrites is impaired in TRPC2 mutant mice: mechanism of pheromone transduction. Neuron 40:551–561
6. Spehr J, Hagendorf S, Weiss J, Spehr M, Leinders-Zufall T, Zufall F (2009) Ca^{2+}-calmodulin feedback mediates sensory adaptation and inhibits pheromone-sensitive ion channels in the vomeronasal organ. J Neurosci 29: 2125–2135
7. Chamero P, Weiss J, Alonso MT, Rodriguez-Prados M, Hisatsune C, Mikoshiba K, Leinders-Zufall T, Zufall F (2017) Type 3 inositol 1,4,5-trisphosphate receptor is dispensable for sensory activation of the mammalian vomeronasal organ. Sci Rep 7:10260
8. Frank JA, Yushchenko DA, Hodson DJ, Lipstein N, Nagpal J, Rutter GA, Rhee JS, Gottschalk A, Brose N, Schultz C, Trauner D (2016) Photoswitchable diacylglycerols enable optical control of protein kinase C. Nat Chem Biol 12:755–762
9. Leinders-Zufall T, Storch U, Bleymehl K, Mederos YSM, Frank JA, Konrad DB, Trauner D, Gudermann T, Zufall F (2018) PhoDAGs enable optical control of diacylglycerol-sensitive transient receptor potential channels. Cell Chem Biol 25:215–223
10. Leinders-Zufall T, Storch U, Mederos YSM, Ojha NK, Koike K, Gudermann T, Zufall F (2021) A diacylglycerol photoswitching protocol for studying TRPC channel functions in mammalian cells and tissue slices. STAR Protoc 2:100527
11. Omura M, Mombaerts P (2014) Trpc2-expressing sensory neurons in the main olfactory epithelium of the mouse. Cell Rep 8:583–595
12. Omura M, Mombaerts P (2015) Trpc2-expressing sensory neurons in the mouse main olfactory epithelium of type B express the soluble guanylate cyclase Gucy1b2. Mol Cell Neurosci 65:114–124
13. Bleymehl K, Pérez-Gómez A, Omura M, Moreno-Pérez A, Macias D, Bai Z, Johnson RS, Leinders-Zufall T, Zufall F, Mombaerts P (2016) A sensor for low environmental oxygen in the mouse main olfactory epithelium. Neuron 92:1196–1203
14. Koike K, Yoo SJ, Bleymehl K, Omura M, Zapiec B, Pyrski M, Blum T, Khan M, Bai Z, Leinders-Zufall T, Mombaerts P, Zufall F (2021) Danger perception and stress response through an olfactory sensor for the bacterial metabolite hydrogen sulfide. Neuron 109: 2469–2484
15. Blum T, Moreno-Pérez A, Pyrski M, Bufe B, Arifovic A, Weissgerber P, Freichel M, Zufall F, Leinders-Zufall T (2019) Trpc5 deficiency causes hypoprolactinemia and altered function of oscillatory dopamine neurons in the arcuate nucleus. Proc Natl Acad Sci U S A 116:15236–15243
16. Müller M, Niemeyer K, Urban N, Ojha NK, Zufall F, Leinders-Zufall T, Schaefer M, Thorn-Seshold O (2022) BTDAzo: A photoswitchable Trpc5 channel activator. Angew Chem Int Ed 61:e202201565
17. Storch U, Forst AL, Pardatscher F, Erdogmus S, Philipp M, Gregoritza M, Mederos YSM, Gudermann T (2017) Dynamic NHERF interaction with TRPC4/5 proteins is required for channel gating by diacylglycerol. Proc Natl Acad Sci U S A 114:E37–E46
18. Eckstein E, Pyrski M, Pinto S, Freichel M, Vennekens R, Zufall F (2020) Cyclic regulation of Trpm4 expression in female vomeronasal neurons driven by ovarian sex hormones. Mol Cell Neurosci 105:103495
19. Pyrski M, Eckstein E, Schmid A, Bufe B, Weiss J, Chubanov V, Boehm U, Zufall F (2017) Trpm5 expression in the olfactory epithelium. Mol Cell Neurosci 80:75–88
20. Lichtenegger M, Tiapko O, Svobodova B, Stockner T, Glasnov TN, Schreibmayer W, Platzer D, de la Cruz GG, Krenn S, Schober R, Shrestha N, Schindl R, Romanin C, Groschner K (2018) An optically controlled probe identifies lipid-gating fenestrations within the TRPC3 channel. Nat Chem Biol 14:396–404
21. Leinders-Zufall T, Lane AP, Puche AC, Ma W, Novotny MV, Shipley MT, Zufall F (2000) Ultrasensitive pheromone detection by

mammalian vomeronasal neurons. Nature 405: 792–796

22. Trouillet AC, Keller M, Weiss J, Leinders-Zufall T, Birnbaumer L, Zufall F, Chamero P (2019) Central role of G protein Gαi2 and Gαi2$^+$ vomeronasal neurons in balancing territorial and infant-directed aggression of male mice. Proc Natl Acad Sci U S A 116:5135–5143
23. Schauer C, Leinders-Zufall T (2012) Imaging calcium responses in GFP-tagged neurons of hypothalamic mouse brain slices. J Vis Exp: e4213
24. Gurtovenko AA, Anwar J (2007) Modulating the structure and properties of cell membranes: the molecular mechanism of action of dimethyl sulfoxide. J Phys Chem B 111:10453–10460
25. Notman R, Noro M, O'Malley B, Anwar J (2006) Molecular basis for dimethylsulfoxide (DMSO) action on lipid membranes. J Am Chem Soc 128:13982–13983
26. Ojha A, Ojha NK (2021) Excitation light-induced phototoxicity during fluorescence imaging. J Biosci 46:78
27. Ojha NK, Nematian-Ardestani E, Neugebauer S, Borowski B, El-Hussein A, Hoshi T, Leipold E, Heinemann SH (2014) Sodium channels as gateable non-photonic sensors for membrane-delimited reactive species. Biochim Biophys Acta 1838:1412–1419

Chapter 4

Intranasal Pressure Recording for Monitoring Mouse Respiration

Emma Janke, Janardhan P. Bhattarai, and Minghong Ma

Abstract

Respiration is a highly dynamic signal that influences voluntary behaviors including odor sampling and entrains rhythmic activity in the brain. Many techniques exist to record respiration with each exhibiting strengths and drawbacks given the ultimate goals of the respiration recording. Intranasal cannula implantation, coupled with pressure sensor recording, allows for temporal precision and detailed feature extraction of the respiratory waveform. Here we describe the implantation process and necessary recording equipment to effectively conduct intranasal pressure recording of respiration. This is an ideal method for understanding the dynamics of odor sampling in conjunction with olfactory sensory transmission.

Key words Respiration, Breathing, Intranasal pressure, Cannula, Sniffing

1 Introduction

Sniffing facilitates dynamic sampling of the olfactory environment. While an array of methodologies exists to record respiration, each consists of unique strengths and concerns, and the chosen technique must be aligned with the overarching goals of the respiration recording [1]. Respiration recordings may be based on measuring pressure change due to airflow, temperature change, or electrophysiology and include the widely used whole-body plethysmography (WBP) [2, 3], intranasal pressure [4–7], intrathoracic pressure [8], intranasal thermocouple [2, 9, 10], pneumotachograph [11], and electromyogram (EMG) recordings of the diaphragm [12, 13]. Local field potential recordings in the olfactory pathway also reflect respiration frequency, but fidelity may vary under different behavioral contexts [2].

WBP continues to be the standard in the respiration field as it is robust, noninvasive, and ideal for extended or chronic recordings of respiration. While animals in WBP are technically not tethered, behavioral tasks are limited to those that are feasible in small

Bradley J. Goldstein and Hiroaki Matsunami (eds.), *The Olfactory System*, Methods in Molecular Biology, vol. 2710, https://doi.org/10.1007/978-1-0716-3425-7_4,

chambers, and breathing signal may be sensitive to motion artifacts occurring during high activity. Intranasal pressure recordings were adapted from head-fixed mice [5] to freely exploring animals [4] to allow for more flexibility in behavioral tests to be investigated. Direct access to respiration within the nasal cavity enables precise alignment of neural responses to inhalation timing and phase where peak contact of odorants with the olfactory epithelium occurs. Evaluating olfactory transmission through a lens of respiration has elicited invaluable information about temporal dynamics of olfactory processing. Furthermore, given intranasal pressure elucidates a detailed respiratory waveform, intranasal pressure recordings have also revealed strong coordination between respiration phase and ultrasonic vocalizations [14].

Here we outline reproducible implantation of intranasal cannulas into the mouse nasal cavity. We also include a list of necessary recording equipment and a suggested BreathMetrics analysis package [15] to simplify the implementation of intranasal pressure recordings.

2 Materials

2.1 Surgery Equipment

1. Stereotaxic apparatus for mouse (68537, RWD).
2. Anesthesia Vaporizer (R583S, RWD) (*see* **Note 1**).
3. Heating pad; preferred self-regulating with rectal probe (*see* **Note 1**).
4. Shaver.
5. Forceps.
6. Dissecting scissors.
7. Sterile cotton applicators.
8. Microdrill (78001, RWD).
9. Drill burr (19007-05 and 19007-09 Fine Science Tools).
10. Self-tapping stainless steel screws (19010-10, Fine Science Tools).
11. Small screwdriver to drive self-tapping screws mentioned above.
12. Intranasal cannula which fits with appropriate dummy cannula (C311G/SPC, P1 Technologies; *see* **Note 2**).
13. 3 M Vetbond adhesive (World Precision Instruments) or Krazy Glue (cyanoacrylate glue).
14. Dental cement and solvent (methyl methacrylate, Cold Cure).
15. Petri dishes (for mixing elastomer and dental cement).
16. Pipette tips (for mixing elastomer and dental cement).

2.2 Animal Care: Pre- and Postoperative Needs

1. Eye lubricant.
2. Vaseline.
3. Ethanol (70% in double distilled water).
4. Povidone-iodine topical aqueous solution (10%).
5. Insulin syringes.
6. Meloxicam.
7. Bupivacaine.
8. Buprenorphine.

2.3 Recording Equipment and Analysis

1. Pressure sensor (CPXL04GF, Honeywell).
2. Soldering system.
3. Power source for pressure sensor, 2.5 V (a Computer USB based cable, split cable to +/− wires with a voltage divider circuit for 5 V; *see* **Note 3**).
4. BNC cable (split to +/− alligator clips to collect respiratory signal from pressure sensor).
5. Cannula collar (303C, P1 Technologies).
6. Cannula tubing PE 20, (C315CT, P1 Technologies).
7. Silicone tubing (ID: 3 mm, OD: 5 mm; fit snug to pressure sensor male end).
8. C-FLEX tubing (06424–60, Cole-Parmer; or equivalent ID: 0.8 mm, OD: 2.4 mm flexible tubing).
9. Parafilm.
10. Syringe needle (18G).
11. Loctite epoxy.
12. Single channel differential amplifier (DP-301, Warner Instruments).
13. Acquisition system (RZ5P Processor and Synapse Software from Tucker-Davis Technologies or other similar systems) to obtain digitized respiratory signal often in conjunction with other signals (i.e., electrophysiology, fiber photometry, and behavioral videos).
14. MATLAB with BreathMetrics analysis package.

3 Methods

3.1 Preoperative Care

1. Sterilize all instruments prior to use.
2. Weigh mouse and calculate proper doses of preoperative injections.

3. Induce deep anesthesia by placing mouse in the chamber at 3% isoflurane.
4. Once mouse is immobile and breathing has slowed, quickly change the anesthesia to the nose cone setting and reduce isoflurane to 1.5–2%.
5. Transfer mouse and position in the stereotaxic apparatus with secured ear bars and nose cone. Ensure that the snout is completely horizontal, i.e., parallel to the surface you are working on (*see* **Note 4**).
6. Shave the dorsal snout and anterior part of the skull behind eyes.
7. Apply eye lubricant to both eyes to prevent drying.
8. Turn on self-regulating heating pad, apply Vaseline to rectal temperature probe, insert, and monitor temperature throughout the procedure.
9. Inject proper doses of preoperative solutions: meloxicam (an anti-inflammatory) subcutaneously and bupivacaine (an analgesic) around incision site on snout.
10. Swab incision area with 10% povidone-iodine followed by 70% ethanol using cotton applicators (complete this process three times).

3.2 Operation

1. Using forceps pinch skin at the midline of the snout and begin incision with dissecting scissors along the midline down to the tip of the nose.
2. Using forceps, open up the incision site to reveal the nasal bones. Using sterile cotton applicators, remove and rub away the transparent membrane over the nasal bone – Fig. 1a shows the exposed nasal bone.
3. Measure 6–8 mm from the tip of the nose and mark where cannula will be implanted (the mark should be at the widest part of the nasal bone which is ~6–8 mm from the tip of the nose). Mark with a sharpie planned placement of the two skull screws. *See* **Note 5**.
4. First drill a hole (drill burr size 0.5 mm; Part No# 19007–05 from Fine Science Tools) for the stabilizing screw #1 – drill slowly, just puncturing the skull to visualize the underlying dura. While drilling, frequently check the fit of the screw into the hole. Once the size of the drilled hole just fits the tip of the screw, screw the end in until just tight and secure with no movement if touched, which can be achieved by turning two to three full-circle twists. *See* **Note 6**.
5. Repeat the procedure for inserting the second screw. Drill the hole and secure the screw into the bone. *See* **Note 7**.

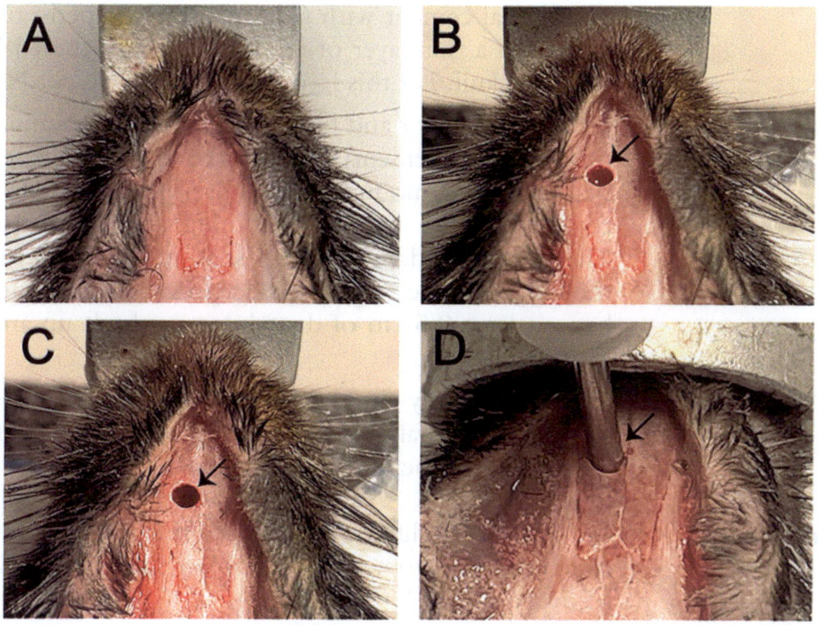

Fig. 1 Implantation of the nasal cannula. (**a**) Dorsal view of the nasal bones after incision. (**b**) Drilled hole prior to cleaning. (**c**) Effective cleaning of the drilled hole prior to cannula insertion. (**d**) Cannula insertion into the nasal cavity

6. Slowly and gently drill the hole (ideally in one touch) for the cannula over the nasal cavity without touching the nasal mucosa. A 0.9 mm drill burr (Part No# 19007–09 from Fine Science Tools) is used because the outside diameter of the cannula C311G is about 1 mm. Underneath the nasal bone, you will begin to view the highly vascular, opaque nasal mucosa (Fig. 1b). After checking that the end of the cannula tightly fits into the hole, proceed to next step. *See* **Note 8.**
7. Puncture the nasal mucosa and clear away any membrane within the hole (Fig. 1c). *See* **Note 9.**
8. Round out the edges of the drilled hole and insert the cannula and adjust the cannula at an angle of ~60 degree from the nasal bone (the top of the cannula slants towards the brain) (Fig. 1d). This angle ensures more uniform airflow to and from the pressure sensor between exhalation and inhalation. *See* **Note 10.**
9. Apply a thin layer of Vetbond or thickened Krazy Glue to the entirety of exposed skull. Vetbond is thin but dries quickly. Krazy Glue should be dispensed onto a petri dish first and given a moment to dry and thicken before application. Either sealant used should be completely dry (not tacky) before moving to the next step.

10. Mix dental cement with solvent using a pipette tip in a petri dish. Add a thin layer of the mixture onto the entirety of the exposed skull. Let this layer cure completely. *See* **Note 11**.
11. Mix more cement and build up around the cannula with multiple layers of cement. Smooth the dental cement out to the base creating a mound on the nose. Allow these layers to cure completely with cement becoming very hard to the touch. These layers of dental cement should extend up to about half the height of the white cannula pedestal. The implant should have at least 0.5 cm of dental cement built up around it (*see* **Note 12**).
12. Once completely cured, take forceps, and pull the skin up the sides of the dental cement. Dab some Vetbond on the inside of the skin and adhere it to the cement.

3.3 Postoperative Care

1. Turn off the isoflurane and remove the mouse from the stereotaxic apparatus to a fresh cage placed on the heating pad for recovery.
2. Inject buprenorphine subcutaneously for postoperative comfort.
3. Follow your lab's protocol for monitoring the animals postoperatively.
4. The mouse should recover for at least a week prior to removing the dummy cannula for recording (*see* **Note 13**).

3.4 Recording and Analysis

1. Follow your manual's instructions for connecting the hardware of the recording acquisition system properly.
2. Refer to Fig. 2 to visualize how to set up a running circuit for a pressure sensor in the lab.
3. Refer to the diagram (Fig. 3) to create a customized connector that screws onto the intranasal cannula for conducting pressure recordings. This connector helps to reduce artifacts caused by repetitive head movements (such as grooming and odor investigation) or by mechanical forces when the mouse bumps into objects/walls. The listed C-FLEX tubing size serves as an ideal attachment, fitting both the top of the intranasal cannula and the suggested cannula tubing. Next, permanently secure the necessary length of cannula tubing (depending on the recording configuration; typically <75 cm) to a small piece (1 cm) of silicone tubing using epoxy and seal with parafilm. This small piece of tubing is then fastened to the end of the pressure sensor.
4. Determine the directionality of your system before performing any recording. Instead of connecting the end of the cannula tube to a mouse with an intranasal cannula, connect a sealed

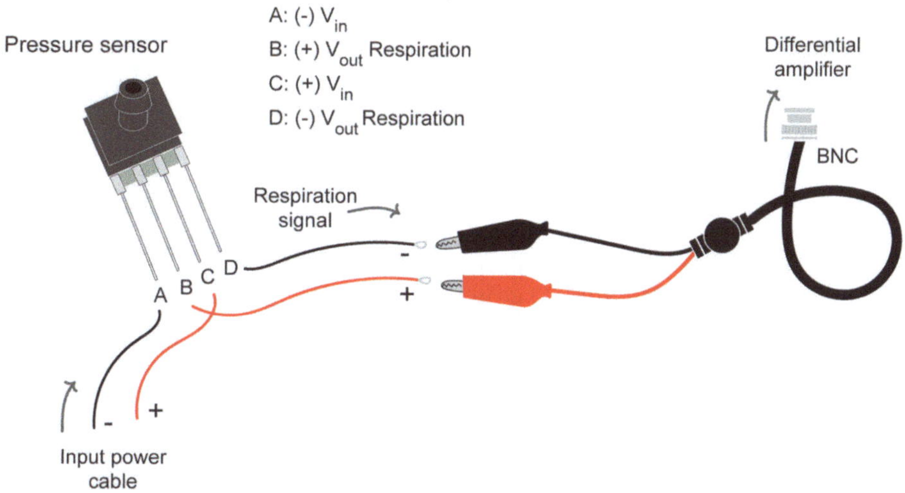

Fig. 2 Schematic demonstrating the setup of a pressure sensor (CPXL04GF, Honeywell) circuit for acquisition of intranasal breathing signal. Connections to the four pins on the pressure sensor are soldered in place

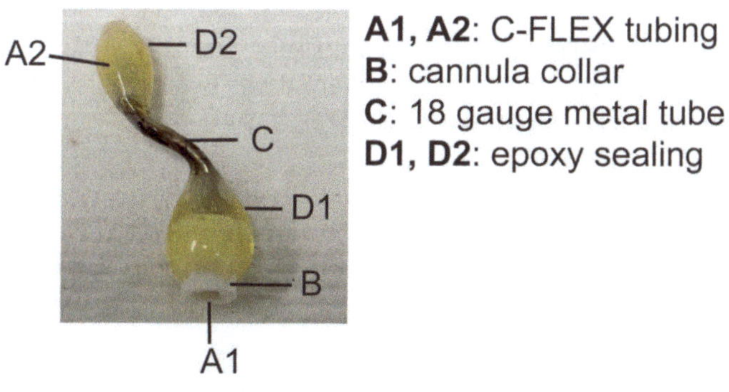

Fig. 3 Image of the connector. C-FLEX tubing is first secured inside a cannula collar with epoxy. A small 18-gauge metal tube is bent and fit into the C-FLEX tubing in the cannula collar. This juncture is sealed with epoxy. The top end of the metal tube is fit with another small piece of C-FLEX tubing and epoxied

syringe. Puff in a small volume of air to the pressure sensor. This air puff mimics an exhale in the nasal cavity by pushing air up to the pressure sensor, so whatever direction this air puff-induced signal goes (positive or negative in the acquisition system) will be the direction of the exhale.

5. Many methods exist to analyze respiration data. An advantage of pressure-based respiration recordings is the ability to detect additional features besides frequency and amplitude. For these nuanced components, we recommend implementing BreathMetrics (Fig. 4). Before using BreathMetrics, ensure the directionality of your recordings matches the orientation in BreathMetrics. Using the 'rodentAirflow' setting in BreathMetrics, inhale is upward. If your recording shows inhale

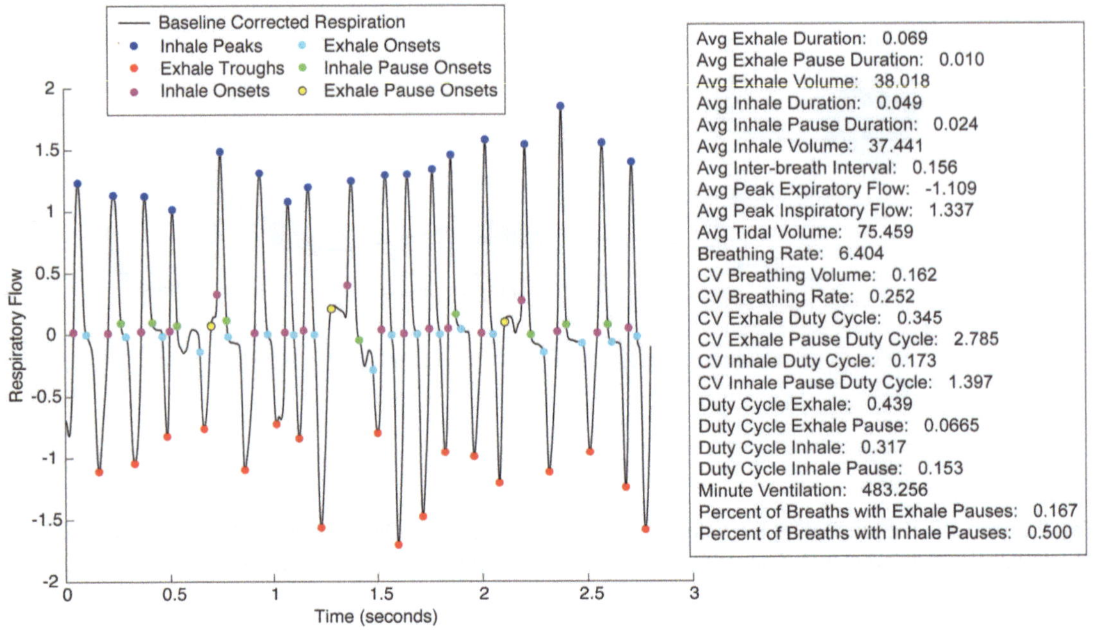

Fig. 4 A representative trace of labelled features in pressure sensor respiratory data using BreathMetrics. The right panel displays 24 quantitative parameters easily extracted with BreathMetrics and highlights the range of information gathered from pressure sensor recordings of respiration

downward, take the inverse of the respiration (multiply the trace by −1) before implementing BreathMetrics. Alternatively, you can change the polarity of the output voltage of the pressure sensor, so that inhale would be upward in your recording.

4 Notes

1. It is preferred to perform cannula implantation under adjustable and well-monitored inhaled isoflurane anesthesia via a nose cone. Intraperitoneal injections of anesthetic mixtures such as ketamine and xylazine have been used and are feasible given the relatively short length of the procedure once mastered. It is highly recommended to implement a self-regulating heating pad during the surgery.
2. C311G corresponds to the guide cannula part number. To prevent it from clogging, a dummy cannula (C311DC) that tightly fits the guide cannula is also required. We implant the intranasal guide cannula with the dummy cannula screwed tightly in place. Cannulas are customizable to needs and animal size. We suggest using C311G that is cut 5 mm below the pedestal and C311DC ordered to fit the 5 mm cannula with a

0.3 mm projection. Once the cap is removed during recording, it leaves enough space for the air flow without getting clogged by mucus. We also suggest removing 1 mm of the white plastic screw from the upper end of the guide cannula prior to the surgery so that it fits perfectly with the C-FLEX tubing inside the connector screw (A2 in Fig. 3) during the respiration recording.

3. Using a USB cable as the power source for the pressure sensor has several advantages: direct connection to the computer, elimination of an additional power supply unit, noise reduction in the recording system, and easy availability of the working voltage. The voltage is reduced from 5 V to ~2.5 V using two identical resistors (<100 Ω) connected in series with the circuit and the positive voltage is drawn from the junction of the two resistors.

4. Throughout the procedure, anesthesia depth must be monitored frequently and especially prior to painful stimuli such as incisions and drilling. Assess the toe pinch reflex, and adjust isoflurane percentage between 1.5–2% or nose cone adjustment if a reaction exists. Monitor the mouse's posture and respiration rate – posture should be relaxed with deep, regular respiration. Shallow, high-frequency respiration tends to indicate too light of anesthesia, and gasping typically reflects hypoxia and too much exposure to isoflurane.

5. Screws are solely for stability and do not require precise coordinates. We recommend one screw be placed slightly posterior to the frontonasal suture, so that it does not obstruct the field of view during cannula implantation. The other screw is placed slightly posterior to the coronal suture. The actual positions of these two screws can be adjusted depending on other implantation(s) on the same mouse (e.g., optical fiber).

6. Self-tapping screws minimize damage and do not require large holes for secure insertion. A small hole that is enough to fit the tip of the screw will suffice as the screw will make its way when being turned and will be very firm. It should be noted that the screw should not be turned more than three full circles as it may damage the brain underneath. Intranasal cannula implantation success depends on the security and sealing of the cannula. Inserting screws first will minimize any potential movement from drilling or inserting screws after cannula insertion.

7. Depending on the angle of the microscope you prefer to view during surgery, you may wait to secure the screw that is ipsilateral to intranasal cannula. This will keep your view open for cannula drilling. The final screw can be secured after cannula implantation and prior to dental cementing.

8. Drilling the hole for the cannula is a critical stage of the procedure. If a 0.9 mm burr is not available to drill the cannula hole in a single touch, the use of a smaller drill burr works but requires slow, careful drilling. In this case, drill a hole the size of the burr and insert the burr back into the hole, drilling outward in slow concentric circles. Frequently check the fit of the cannula to the hole in progress. If the hole is drilled too quickly and becomes too large for the cannula, it is challenging to correct. If the size of the hole is just slightly off, sometimes corrections can be made by packing around the cannula with bone wax to make the fit tighter. Overall, the cannula should snugly fit into the hole in the nasal bone with no movement when touched or open space for leaks.
9. There are many methods to puncture the nasal mucosa. Lightly touching the nasal mucosa with the powered-on drill can create the first puncture. Less risky alternatives include using an insulin syringe to puncture the mucosa. The mucosa will almost always bleed while freeing space to insert the cannula. Tightly twist a Kim Wipe's corner to make an absorbent wand and insert it into the hole to absorb the blood. Start with a small puncture to ensure you see the dark open space of the nasal cavity underneath. Clearing away the nasal mucosa is another crucial stage that impacts success of implantation. Always use gentle, small movements. Be careful to ensure the nasal mucosa stays in place dorsally while clearing and that you are not pushing the mucosa down into the nasal cavity. If using the insulin syringe method, you will have to continue to probe the puncture with a twisted Kim Wipe and/or syringe to open up the hole in the tissue to allow for insertion of the cannula. Ideally you should not have mucosa blocking any part of the hole for the cannula as the tissue may regenerate and block the cannula.
10. For cannula insertion, ideally the edge of the guide cannula will be flush with the nasal bone, and the projection of the dummy cannula protrudes into the nasal cavity to block where the tissue may regenerate. One way to track depth of guide cannula insertion into the nasal cavity is by marking the edge of guide cannula with a dark marker. This provides a reference for cannula depth based upon how much remainder of the marked ring you can view once inserted.
11. For the first layer of dental cement, keep the mixed solution thinner so that it binds and smooths well across the skull. Following layers of dental cement that build up around the cannula may be added when the mixture is thicker.

12. Take care to not accidentally cement too close to the dummy cannula top. Space must be left to fit a connecting tube to the pressure sensor.
13. The intranasal cannula may cause some inflammation. Mice tend to adapt well, but you may find that mice need to sneeze out some congestion and show poor or noisy respiratory signal on the first recording day. If animals continue to show poor signal, you may slowly puff a small volume of air into the cannula to help clear. This must be done cautiously as a large volume of air, too forcefully may damage the lungs and be lethal or potentially dislodge the cannula. Alternatively, you may irrigate the cannula with saline at a very slow rate and allow mice to sneeze out the saline.
14. Intranasal cannulas and screws are reusable. Head caps can be removed and soaked in acetone to soften and remove the dental cement from parts.

Acknowledgments

This work was supported by the National Institutes of Health R01DC006213 to M.M., R21DC019193 to J.P.B., and F31MH124372 to E.J.

References

1. Grimaud J, Murthy VN (2018) How to monitor breathing in laboratory rodents: a review of the current methods. J Neurophysiol 120:624–632
2. Jessberger J, Zhong W, Brankack J, Draguhn A (2016) Olfactory Bulb Field Potentials and Respiration in Sleep-Wake States of Mice. Neural Plast 2016:4570831
3. Wesson DW, Varga-Wesson AG, Borkowski AH, Wilson DA (2011) Respiratory and sniffing behaviors throughout adulthood and aging in mice. Behav Brain Res 223:99–106
4. Wesson DW, Donahou TN, Johnson MO, Wachowiak M (2008) Sniffing behavior of mice during performance in odor-guided tasks. Chem Senses 33:581–596
5. Verhagen JV, Wesson DW, Netoff TI, White JA, Wachowiak M (2007) Sniffing controls an adaptive filter of sensory input to the olfactory bulb. Nat Neurosci 10:631–639
6. Smear M, Shusterman R, O'Connor R, Bozza T, Rinberg D (2011) Perception of sniff phase in mouse olfaction. Nature 479: 397–400
7. Shusterman R, Smear MC, Koulakov AA, Rinberg D (2011) Precise olfactory responses tile the sniff cycle. Nat Neurosci 14:1039–1044
8. Reisert J, Golden GJ, Matsumura K, Smear M, Rinberg D, Gelperin A (2014) Comparing thoracic and intra-nasal pressure transients to monitor active odor sampling during odor-guided decision making in the mouse. J Neurosci Methods 221:8–14
9. McAfee SS, Ogg MC, Ross JM, Liu Y, Fletcher ML, Heck DH (2016) Minimally invasive highly precise monitoring of respiratory rhythm in the mouse using an epithelial temperature probe. J Neurosci Methods 263:89–94
10. Schreck MR, Zhuang L, Janke E, Moberly AH, Bhattarai JP, Gottfried JA, Wesson DW, Ma M (2022) State-dependent olfactory processing in freely behaving mice. Cell Rep 38:110450
11. Youngentob SL, Mozell MM, Sheehe PR, Hornung DE (1987) A quantitative analysis of sniffing strategies in rats performing odor detection tasks. Physiol Behav 41:59–69

12. Herent C, Diem S, Fortin G, Bouvier J (2020) Absent phasing of respiratory and locomotor rhythms in running mice. elife 9
13. Rojas-Libano D, Frederick DE, Egana JI, Kay LM (2014) The olfactory bulb theta rhythm follows all frequencies of diaphragmatic respiration in the freely behaving rat. Front Behav Neurosci 8:214
14. Sirotin YB, Costa ME, Laplagne DA (2014) Rodent ultrasonic vocalizations are bound to active sniffing behavior. Front Behav Neurosci 8:399
15. Noto T, Zhou G, Schuele S, Templer J, Zelano C (2018) Automated analysis of breathing waveforms using BreathMetrics: a respiratory signal processing toolbox. Chem Senses 43: 583–597

Chapter 5

Identification of Immune Cells in Murine Olfactory Mucosa

Sebastian A. Wellford and E. Ashley Moseman

Abstract

Olfactory immunology is an emerging field in the context of infectious disease and neuroimmunology, yet characterization of immune cells within the murine olfactory mucosa remains sparse. This is partially due to the difficulty in distinguishing olfactory-resident immune cells from immune cells that reside within nasal turbinate bone marrow. Using techniques like intranasal antibody labeling, we have developed methods to definitively identify olfactory immune cells via flow cytometry and immunofluorescent confocal microscopy. This protocol will describe the best practices for these methods, as well as detail how intravenous antibody labeling can be used to study the blood-olfactory barrier, an important determinant of olfactory immunity. We also include validated markers for the identification of major olfactory immune populations.

Key words Olfactory immunology, Mucosal immunity, Neuroimmunology, Intranasal antibody labeling, Flow cytometry, Immunofluorescent confocal microscopy, Blood-olfactory barrier

1 Introduction

The olfactory mucosa is increasingly recognized as an important immune tissue, both as an impediment against CNS olfactory neuroinvasion and as a major component of the upper respiratory barrier [1–9]. Therefore, analysis of the tissue-resident immune cells in the olfactory mucosa is relevant to ongoing studies of infectious disease and neuroimmunity. Identification of olfactory immune cells is complicated by nasal turbinate anatomy [10, 11]. The olfactory mucosa rests on bony turbinates that contain numerous $CD45^+$ immune cells. Digestion of the olfactory mucosa to form single-cell suspensions requires mincing of the nasal turbinates, overwhelming the bona fide olfactory immune cells with bone marrow contaminate. Herein, we describe the methods we have developed to identify and analyze tissue-resident immune cells of the olfactory mucosa in mice.

This chapter will describe procedures for the identification of olfactory immune cells by flow cytometry, the visualization of olfactory immune cells by immunofluorescent histochemistry, and

Bradley J. Goldstein and Hiroaki Matsunami (eds.), *The Olfactory System*, Methods in Molecular Biology, vol. 2710,
https://doi.org/10.1007/978-1-0716-3425-7_5,

the examination of the blood-olfactory barrier. Each of these procedures provides an improved methodology for the study of olfactory immunology. Intranasal labeling prior to the formation of single-cell suspensions enables the study of olfactory-resident immune cells, as opposed to contaminating immune cells from nasal turbinate bone marrow. These single-cell suspensions can be used for conventional flow cytometry, as well as for methods including single-cell RNA sequencing. A reliable procedure for immunofluorescent confocal microscopy allows for imaging of extravascular olfactory immune cells while maintaining nasal turbinate structure. Lastly, our protocol for intravenous antibody labeling can be used to assess integrity of the recently discovered blood-olfactory barrier (BOB) [2]. The BOB prevents circulating antibody from accessing the olfactory mucosa, dramatically impacting immunity at the mucosal barrier. If the BOB is compromised, intravenous antibody will leak into the olfactory mucosa. Together, these methods will advance studies of murine olfactory immunology and infectious disease.

2 Materials

2.1 Generation of Olfactory Mucosa Single-Cell Suspensions for Flow Cytometry

1. Scissors.
2. Forceps.
3. 20 mL syringe and 20 gauge needle.
4. Institutionally approved method to achieve a surgical plane of anesthesia (injectables are the most practical).
5. PBS.
6. 24-well plate.
7. Tissue Digest: hibernate A w/ DNAse (0.5 mg/mL) and collagenase (0.5 mg/mL). Hibernate A is used to preserve neuronal health, other media types may work for your application.
8. Pipette and tips.
9. 5 ml 12x 75 mm polystyrene tubes (5 mL tube).
10. Trypan Blue.
11. Formalin-buffered phosphate fixative: 10% buffered formalin, diluted to 1.25% with PBS, can also use any other flow cytometry compatible fixative.

2.2 Immunofluorescent Histochemistry of Olfactory Mucosa

1. 2.5% formalin-buffered phosphate fixative: 10% buffered formalin, diluted to 2.5% with PBS, can also use 2.5% freshly prepared paraformaldehyde solution.
2. 20 mL syringe and 20 gauge needle.
3. Institutionally approved method to achieve a surgical plane of anesthesia (injectables are the most practical).

4. Scissors.
5. 50 mL conical tube.
6. 2 mL serological pipette and vacuum line.
7. 0.5 M EDTA.
8. Razor blade.
9. Tissue Freezing Media (General Data, TFM-5).
10. Cryomold Standard (Tissue-Tek).
11. Cryostat.
12. Microscope slides (FisherBrand SuperFrost Plus).
13. Mounting media: 774 μM Mowiol 4–88, 0.65 M glycerol, 67% Tris–HCl (0.2 M pH 8.5), 2.5% DABCO 33-LV.
14. Cover slips.

2.3 Intravenous Antibody labeling

1. α-EpCAM antibody (G8.8).
2. α-Rat IgG-AlexaFluor647 secondary antibody (Poly4054, Biolegend).

3 Methods

3.1 Generation of Olfactory Mucosa Single-Cell Suspensions for Flow Cytometry

1. Anesthetize mice by your institutionally approved sedation to achieve a surgical plane of anesthesia. Ensure the lack of animal reflexes before proceeding. Insufficient anesthesia will cause the animal distress and result in expulsion of your intranasally administered antibody.
2. Intranasal antibody labeling: To distinguish CD45+ cells of the olfactory mucosa from cells in the bone marrow for flow cytometry, intranasally label with α-CD45.2 antibody. Pipette 5 μL onto each nare of the mouse nostril and allow the mouse to inhale the droplet. Wait no more than 5 min before proceeding to perfusion. See Fig. 1a–d for intranasal CD45 staining.
3. Perform intracardiac perfusion of the mouse using the needle and syringe with 5–10 mL of PBS. Perfusion reduces the number of circulating leukocytes in the sample and makes tissue dissection more convenient by reducing blood volume in the nasal turbinates.
4. To harvest the olfactory mucosa, first remove the brain. Use scissors to make an incision on the back of the neck of the mouse. Peel the skin off the skull of the mouse. Puncture the interparietal bone in the back, soft part of the skull with the scissors. Make incisions along both sides of the head, all the way down to the frontonasal suture at the bridge of the nose. Remove the skullcap and then the brain. Use forceps to pry off the nasal bones, grasping from the nose tip (this will expose two long openings into the nasal cavity). Using two forceps,

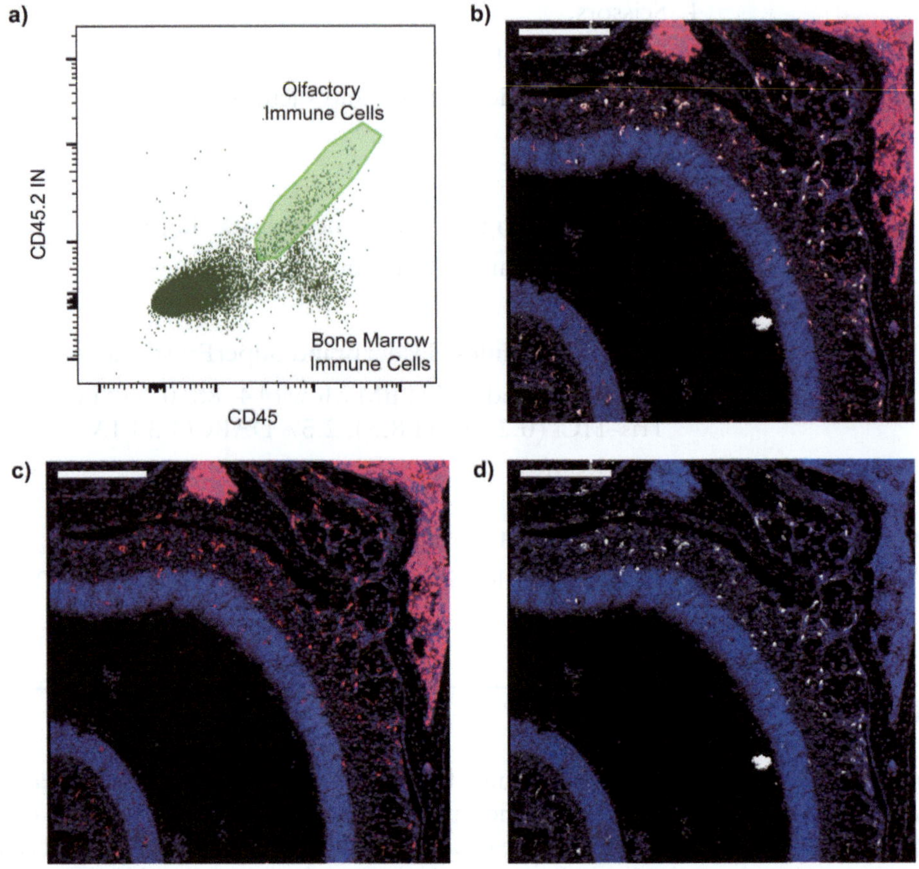

Fig. 1 Intranasal labeling of OM immune cells. Demonstration of how intranasal antibody labeling can distinguish olfactory mucosa immune cells from immune cells within nasal turbinate bone marrow. (**a**) Flow cytometry of digested OM tissue stained intranasally with α-CD45.2 antibody, followed by conventional α-CD45 after digest. Gate highlights double-positive olfactory immune cells. (**b–d**) Confocal microscopy of $CD45^+$ cells in the olfactory mucosa. Prior to sacrifice, α-CD45.2 antibody was administered IN. Olfactory immune cells are $CD45^+/CD45.2^+$, while bone marrow cells are $CD45^+/CD45.2^-$. (**b**) Merged image, (**c**) CD45 only, (**d**) CD45.2 IN only. Blue, DAPI; white, IN CD45.2; red, CD45; scale bar, 200 μm

separate the premaxilla bones, exposing the nasal turbinates. Lift out the olfactory tissue with the forceps, which should be a yellow, mucosal tissue. Remove any remaining turbinate pieces. The lateral nasal glands ("soft," white, flat, and round tissues) may cling to both sides of the turbinates, these should be peeled out and removed from the collected turbinates.

5. Place the olfactory turbinates in a 24-well plate with 0.5 mL of the Tissue Digest in each well (*see* **Note 1**). Mince the tissue using small scissors. Digest at 37 °C with 600 rpm shaking for 30 min (*see* **Note 2**).
6. Transfer the digested tissues to 5 mL round bottom tubes. Add 3 mL PBS and centrifuge at 400× *g* for 5 min. Aspirate or pour off the supernatant without disrupting the cell pellet.

7. Resuspend the cells in 1 mL PBS. Take 10 μL to count cells using Trypan Blue exclusion or similar counting dye. Prepare an antibody staining cocktail at the desired antibody concentrations. See Table 1 for useful OM immune cell markers. Spin down cells at 400× *g* for 5 min, and resuspend in 200 μL of the antibody staining cocktail. Stain at room temperature for 15 min or at 4 degrees Celsius for 30 min.

8. Wash cells with PBS and fix in 1.25% formalin-buffered phosphate, if desired, for flow cytometry.

Table 1
Useful olfactory mucosa immune cell markers

Antibody (application) [clone]	Cell type
α-CD45 (flow cytometry, IF) [30-F11]	Hematopoietic cells
α-CD45.2 (flow cytometry, IF) [104]	Hematopoietic cells
α-CD11b (flow cytometry) [M1/70]	Myeloid cells
α-Gr-1 (flow cytometry, IF) [RB6/8C5]	Neutrophils/monocytes
α-Ly6g (flow cytometry, IF) [1A8]	Neutrophils
α-Ly6c (flow cytometry) [HK1.4]	Monocytes
α-Cx3cr1 (flow cytometry) [QA16A03]	Monocytes/macrophages
α-F4/80 (flow cytometry, IF) [BM8]	Macrophages
α-CD64 (flow cytometry, IF) [X54–5/7.1]	Macrophages
α-CD11c (flow cytometry) [N418]	Dendritic cells
α-IA/IE (flow cytometry, IF) [M5/114.15.2]	Dendritic cells, macrophages
α-CD3 (flow cytometry) [17A2]	T cells
α-Thy1.2 (flow cytometry) [53–2.1]	T cells
α-Tcrβ (flow cytometry, IF) [H57–597]	αβ T cells
α-CD4 (flow cytometry) [RM4–5]	CD4+ T cells
α-CD8a (flow cytometry, IF) [53–6.7]	CD8+ T cells, dendritic cells
α-CD19 (flow cytometry) [6D5]	B cells
α-CD45R/B220 (flow cytometry, IF) [RA3-6B2]	B cells
α-CD138 (IF)* [281–2]	Plasma cells
α-NK1.1 (flow cytometry) [PK136]	NK cells
α-SiglecF (flow cytometry) [S17007L]	Eosinophils

These markers are validated for each indicated method to identify immune cells within the olfactory mucosa. IF, immunofluorescent confocal microscopy. *CD138 (Syndecan-1) is cleaved by the Tissue Digest and therefore cannot be used for flow cytometry

3.2 Immunofluorescent Histochemistry of Olfactory Mucosa

1. Anesthetize mice by intraperitoneal (i.p.) injection of your institutionally approved sedation to achieve a surgical plane of anesthesia.
2. Perform intracardiac perfusion of the mouse using the needle and syringe with 5–10 mL of 2.5% formalin-buffered phosphate fixative (*see* **Note 3**). Use scissors to remove the head, as well as the lower jaw to allow for easier decalcification and sectioning.
3. *Optional:* for whole mount imaging of olfactory tissue, peel the septum tissue from the nasal cavity as described previously [12].
4. Submerge the head in 2.5% fixative, and degas the sample to remove air from the nasal cavity and ensure good fixative contact. Degassing can be done by puncturing a hole in the top of the 50 mL conical tube large enough to insert a 2 mL serological pipette attached to a vacuum line. Turn on the vacuum line for 5 min, thereby removing bubbles from the nasal cavity of the mouse. Keep the head in 2.5% formalin at room temperature for 3 hours. Transfer the heads, still submerged in fixative, into a 4 °C fridge overnight.
5. Remove the fixative from the tube. Submerge the heads in 0.5 M EDTA for decalcification. Place the heads in the 4 °C fridge for 5 days to allow for full decalcification (*see* **Note 4**).
6. Embed the tissues in Tissue Freezing Media at the desired orientation for sectioning (*see* **Note 5**). For coronal sections, which provide the best view of olfactory turbinates (see Fig. 1b–d), use a razor to bisect the head just rostral of the olfactory bulb at the bridge of the nose. Angle the razor slightly down (~20°) toward the bottom/back of the head to go through olfactory tissue that extends beneath the olfactory bulb. Blot any excess liquid from tissue, then place the two pieces of tissue, cut side down, in Tissue Freezing Media (TFM) in a standard histology cassette (remove any excess tissue that doesn't fit in the cassette). For sagittal sections, which provide a simultaneous view of the respiratory and olfactory epithelia, as well as the olfactory bulb, use a razor to cut the head in half 1–2 mm from the midline (to avoid disrupting the septum). Place the flat sides of both tissues down in TFM in a histology cassette. For axial sections, which provide a view of the olfactory epithelium and olfactory bulb, the entire head can be placed into the TFM-filled cryomold with the dorsal surface at the cryomold bottom. Freeze and store embedded tissues at −80 °C for long-term storage. Storage at −25 °C will result in TFM dessication, and sectioning will be very difficult.
7. To make cryosections, use a cryostat set to −15 to −22 °C (*see* **Note 6**). Section thickness of 30 microns allows for stable

turbinate structure and imaging of multiple layers of cells, but sections can be made as thin as 5 microns. Adhere sections directly to microscope slide.

8. To stain tissue sections directly on the slide, wash with PBS, stain with antibody overnight at 4 °C or at room temperature for 4 hours, and wash with PBS (*see* **Note** 7). Repeat with secondary stain if required. Add droplets of mounting media (Mowiol [13], or similar media), and lay coverslip over tissue. See Table 1 for useful markers for olfactory immune cells and olfactory structures.
9. Image tissues on immunofluorescent confocal microscope.

3.3 Intravenous Antibody Labeling

1. Intravenously inject 20 μg α-EpCAM in 100 μl of sterile PBS 12 h prior to sacrificing the mouse. α-EpCAM can be reliably detected in peripheral tissues 4–24 h following injection, but signal intensity peaks around 12 h.
2. Perfuse mouse with fixative, and prepare sections for immunofluorescent confocal microscopy as above. Sagittal sections allow for simultaneous visualization of juxtaposed olfactory and respiratory epithelia,
3. Use secondary α-Rat IgG antibody to stain for α-EpCAM. As an ex vivo staining control, take serial sections and stain with ex vivo α-EpCAM primary antibody followed by secondary α-Rat IgG stain.

4 Notes

1. More aggressive tissue digests can be used to dissociate endothelial cells or a greater number of immune cells. For example, Hibernate A with Collagenase P and Dispase I can more completely digest the mucosa. However, these digests will cause loss of cell surface markers, and conditions should be tested with controls to determine the degree of loss.
2. Pipette the digested tissue up and down during and after the shaking procedure to help achieve a more complete digestion.
3. 2.5% formalin-buffered phosphate fixative is superior to 4%; the lower fixative concentration allows for less background autofluorescence, greater epitope preservation, and a broader range of antibodies to bind their targets. This also prevents brittle nasal bones from fracturing due to overfixation.
4. Periodically inverting the tube can accelerate the decalcification process. Heads should slice easily with little resistance from bone. If resistance or "crunching" occurs, place the tissue back in EDTA for additional decalcification.

5. In our hands, Tissue Freezing Media outperforms O.C.T. (optimal cutting temperature) for preparing thick olfactory mucosa sections (~30 microns). Formulation changes to commercially available TFM have recently made sectioning more challenging.
6. Optimal cryostat sectioning temperature needs to be empirically determined based on the instrument, room airflow, and user preference. Keep embedded tissues at −15 °C only for short periods of time (<4 h) to avoid dessication. Store at −80 °C for long-term preservation.
7. To find the optimal antibody concentration for staining olfactory sections directly on the slide, use roughly twice the concentration one would use for flow cytometry.

Acknowledgments

E.A.M. is partially supported by 1R01NS121067, 1R21AG074324, and by the Duke School of Medicine Whitehead Family Scholarship. S.A.W. received support from T32AI052077.

References

1. Dumm RE, Wellford SA, Moseman EA, Heaton NS (2020) Heterogeneity of antiviral responses in the upper respiratory tract mediates differential non-lytic clearance of influenza viruses. Cell Rep 32:108103
2. Wellford SA, Moseman AP, Dao K, Wright KE, Chen A, Plevin JE, Liao TC, Mehta N, Moseman EA (2022) Mucosal plasma cells are required to protect the upper airway and brain from infection. Immunity 55(2118–2134):e2116
3. Shivkumar M, Milho R, May JS, Nicoll MP, Efstathiou S, Stevenson PG (2013) Herpes simplex virus 1 targets the murine olfactory neuroepithelium for host entry. J Virol 87:10477–10488
4. Dando SJ, Mackay-Sim A, Norton R, Currie BJ, St John JA, Ekberg JA, Batzloff M, Ulett GC, Beacham IR (2014) Pathogens penetrating the central nervous system: infection pathways and the cellular and molecular mechanisms of invasion. Clin Microbiol Rev 27:691–726
5. Lawler C, Stevenson PG (2017) Type I Interferon Signaling to Dendritic Cells Limits Murid Herpesvirus 4 Spread from the Olfactory Epithelium. J Virol 91:e00951–e00917
6. Ampie L, McGavern DB (2022) Immunological defense of CNS barriers against infections. Immunity 55:781–799
7. Brann DH, Tsukahara T, Weinreb C, Lipovsek M, Van den Berge K, Gong B, Chance R, Macaulay IC, Chou HJ, Fletcher RB et al (2020) Non-neuronal expression of SARS-CoV-2 entry genes in the olfactory system suggests mechanisms underlying COVID-19-associated anosmia. Sci Adv 6. https://doi.org/10.1126/sciadv.abc5801
8. de Melo GD, Lazarini F, Levallois S, Hautefort C, Michel V, Larrous F, Verillaud B, Aparicio C, Wagner S, Gheusi G et al (2021) COVID-19-related anosmia is associated with viral persistence and inflammation in human olfactory epithelium and brain infection in hamsters. Sci Transl Med 13. https://doi.org/10.1126/scitranslmed.abf8396
9. Khan M, Yoo SJ, Clijsters M, Backaert W, Vanstapel A, Speleman K, Lietaer C, Choi S, Hether TD, Marcelis L et al (2021) Visualizing in deceased COVID-19 patients how SARS-CoV-2 attacks the respiratory and olfactory mucosae but spares the olfactory bulb. Cell 184(5932–5949):e5915. https://doi.org/10.1016/j.cell.2021.10.027

10. McEwen DP, Jenkins PM, Martens JR (2008) Olfactory cilia: our direct neuronal connection to the external world. Curr Top Dev Biol 85: 333–370
11. Barrios AW, Nunez G, Sanchez Quinteiro P, Salazar I (2014) Anatomy, histochemistry, and immunohistochemistry of the olfactory subsystems in mice. Front Neuroanat 8:1–10
12. Oberland S, Neuhaus EM (2014) Whole mount labeling of cilia in the main olfactory system of mice. J Vis Exp JoVE. https://doi.org/10.3791/52299
13. Cold Spring Harbor Protocols (2006) Mowiol mounting medium. https://doi.org/10.1101/pdb.rec10255

Chapter 6

Chromatin Immunoprecipitation from Formaldehyde Cross-Linked Olfactory Sensory Neurons

Jerome K. Kahiapo and Kevin Monahan

Abstract

Chromatin immunoprecipitation (ChIP) allows a researcher to determine the genomic occupancy of nuclear proteins, providing insight into the roles of transcription factors, chromatin modifiers, histone modifications, and other factors bound to DNA. Protein-DNA interactions are first fixed in vivo by chemical cross-linking, and then a target protein is captured together with any associated DNA by an antibody mediated pull-down. The co-immunoprecipitated DNA can then be assayed by quantitative PCR or deep sequencing. Here, we demonstrate this technique using murine olfactory sensory neurons (OSNs) purified using fluorescence-activated cell sorting (FACS) and antibodies for the ubiquitous chromatin protein CTCF.

Key words Chromatin, Immunoprecipitation, Formaldehyde, Cross-link, Sonication, CTCF, Olfactory sensory neuron

1 Introduction

Genomic DNA assembles with proteins to form chromatin. The composition and organization of chromatin regulate a multitude of processes including transcription, DNA repair, and the three-dimensional folding of the genome. When studying these processes, it is often important to identify the regions of the genome that are associated with a protein of interest and to determine what the relative occupancy of that protein is across its genomic binding sites. Chromatin immunoprecipitation (ChIP) allows the measurement of genomic occupancy through antibody mediated capture of chromatin-DNA complexes [1, 2]. Protein-DNA complexes are first covalently cross-linked in intact cells using formaldehyde [3]. The fixed cells are lysed, nuclei are purified, and then the nuclear chromatin is sheared into small fragments by sonication. Next, antibodies are used to immunoprecipitate chromatin fragments containing the protein of interest. Finally, the DNA

Bradley J. Goldstein and Hiroaki Matsunami (eds.), *The Olfactory System*, Methods in Molecular Biology, vol. 2710,
https://doi.org/10.1007/978-1-0716-3425-7_6,

fragments that co-immunoprecipitate with the target protein are purified. This ChIP DNA can then be assayed for the presence of specific sites of interest, for example, by quantitative PCR, or it can be prepared into ChIP-seq libraries, which allow the genome-wide identification and quantification of target protein bound sites by deep sequencing [4, 5].

Numerous protocols for chromatin immunoprecipitation ChIP have been described, but these protocols usually require tens of millions of cells and frequently must be adapted when applied to new cell types. Here, we present a ChIP protocol optimized for labeled populations of primary cells purified from the mouse main olfactory epithelium (MOE) by flow cytometry. We have successfully used this protocol to ChIP several proteins, including CTCF, Rad21, Lhx2, Ldb1, and Ebf, from as few as 250,000 cells [6–8]. As an example, we described the ChIP of CTCF from olfactory sensory neurons labeled with OMP-IRES-GFP [9]. We describe the full experimental workflow, including the dissociation of the MOE, the fixation, purification and lysis of labeled cells, the preparation of sonicated chromatin, and finally the ChIP itself. The entire protocol can be completed in as few as 3 days, but we also identify optional stopping points.

2 Materials

All reagents are prepared in nuclease-free water. Filtered pipette tips and DNA low-binding 1.5 mL Eppendorf tubes are used throughout.

2.1 Isolation and Fixation of Dissociated Cells

1. Papain dissociation kit (Worthington Biochemical).
2. Dissection tools.
3. 35 mm glass Petri dish.
4. 40 um nylon filter tubes.
5. Phosphate buffered saline (PBS).
6. Formaldehyde fixation solution: 1% formaldehyde in PBS (*see* **Note 1**).
7. Glycine: 1.25 M glycine solution diluted in water.
8. Sort media: 2% fetal bovine serum in PBS **OR** 1% BSA in PBS.

2.2 Cell Lysis and Chromatin Sonication

1. Covaris ultrasonicator and 130uL AFA shearing vials (*see* **Note 2**).
2. cOmplete EDTA-free Protease Inhibitor Cocktail: dissolve 1 tablet in 500 uL nuclease-free water to make a 100× "Protease Inhibitor Cocktail" stock.

3. Fluorescence-based assay for quantifying the concentration of dsDNA, such as PicoGreen or QuantiFluor.
4. DNA column purification kit.
5. 10 mg/mL RNase A.
6. 20 mg/mL proteinase K.
7. Lysis buffer: 50 mM Tris–HCl pH 7.5, 0.5% Igepal ca-630, 0.25% sodium deoxycholate, 0.1% SDS, 150 mM NaCl. Add Protease Inhibitor Cocktail immediately before use by diluting the100× stock solution.
8. Shearing buffer: 10 mM Tris–HCl pH 7.5, 1 mM EDTA, 0.25% SDS. Add Protease Inhibitor Cocktail immediately before use by diluting the 100× stock solution.

2.3 Chromatin Immunoprecipitation

1. Magnetic rack suitable for 1.5 mL microcentrifuge tubes.
2. Rotary mixer.
3. Thermomixer or similar heat block with shaking (*see* **Note 3**).
4. DNA LoBind 1.5 mL tubes.
5. Protein G Dynabeads.
6. Zymo ChIP DNA Clean & Concentrator kit, or similar.
7. 20 mg/mL Yeast tRNA.
8. 20 mg/mL proteinase K.
9. Anti-CTCF antibody (Millipore 07–729).
10. ChIP Dilution Buffer (CDB): 16.7 mM Tris–HCl pH 7.5, 167 mM NaCl, 1.1% Triton-X 100, 1.2 mM EDTA (with and without Protease Inhibitor Cocktail).
11. Lithium chloride wash solution: 100 mM Tris–HCl pH 7.5, 500 mM LiCl, 1% NP-40, 1% sodium deoxycholate.
12. TE pH 7.5: 10 mM Tris–HCl pH 7.5, 20 mM EDTA.
13. Elution buffer: 100 mM NaHCO3, 1% SDS. Add 5 mM DTT immediately prior to use.

3 Methods

3.1 Isolation and Fixation of Dissociated Cells

1. Prepare papain dissociation solutions from the Worthington papain dissociation kit. Prepare a vial of the albumin ovomucoid inhibitor vial by adding 32 mL of EBSS and incubating, open, in a 37 °C CO_2 incubator for 30 min. This stock can be stored at 4 °C for 3 months. Prepare a vial of papain by adding 5 mL of EBSS, incubate in a 37 °C water bath for 10 min, and then place at room temperature. Prepare a vial of DNase by adding 500 uL EBSS, gently mix, and then place on ice. Prepare 3 mL of diluted albumin ovomucoid inhibitor solution

by adding 300 uL of the inhibitor stock solution to 2.7 mL EBSS, and then place at room temperature (*see* **Note 4**).

2. Euthanize 5 OMP-GFP+ mice following approved euthanasia techniques (*see* **Note 5**). Carefully dissect out the MOEs, and place on ice in a clean glass dish containing 1–2 mL of cold PBS. The number of OMP-GFP+ cells that can be isolated from each mouse is age dependent (*see* **Note 6**).
3. Transfer dissected MOEs to a flat, dry glass dish on ice. Roughly chop the tissue using a clean razor blade.
4. Combine 5 mL of papain with 250 uL of DNase solution in a 15 mL conical tube (*see* **Note 7**). Add the chopped tissue, and incubate on a rotary mixer at 37 °C for 30 min.
5. Triturate the papain treated tissue 20 times with a 5 mL serological pipette, avoiding bubbles. Let sit 1 minute at room temperature to allow large particulates to settle, then transfer the supernatant solution, which contains dissociated cells, to a new 15 mL tube. Using a 1000 uL pipet tip, carefully collect any remaining liquid from the bottom of the tube while leaving large debris behind, and then add it to the supernatant solution.
6. Pellet cells by centrifuging the supernatant solution in a swinging bucket rotor at 300 g for 5 min at room temperature.
7. Discard the supernatant and gently resuspend the cell pellet in 3 mL of the diluted inhibitor solution. Centrifuge again at 300 g for 5 min at room temperature.
8. Discard the supernatant and resuspend the cell pellet with 5 mL of room temperature formaldehyde fixation solution. Incubate on a rotary mixer for 5 min at room temperature (*see* **Note 8**).
9. Quench the fixation reaction by adding 500 uL (1/10 volume) of 1.25 M glycine and rotate for 5 min at room temperature. Pellet the fixed cells by centrifuging at 500 g for 5 min in a pre-cooled 4 °C swinging bucket rotor (*see* **Note 9**).
10. Discard the supernatant in appropriate chemical waste container. Wash cells once by resuspending the pellet in cold sort media, then centrifuge again at 500 g for 5 min at 4 °C.
11. Discard the supernatant, and then resuspend the pellet in 1–2 mL cold sort media (0.2–0.4 mL per MOE). Pass this solution through a 40 um filter to remove debris and clumps (*see* **Note 10**).
12. Purify fixed OMP-GFP+ cells using a fluorescence-activated cell sorter (Fig. 1; *see* **Note 11**). Collect sorted cells in a 15 mL polypropylene conical tubes containing 4 mL sort media.

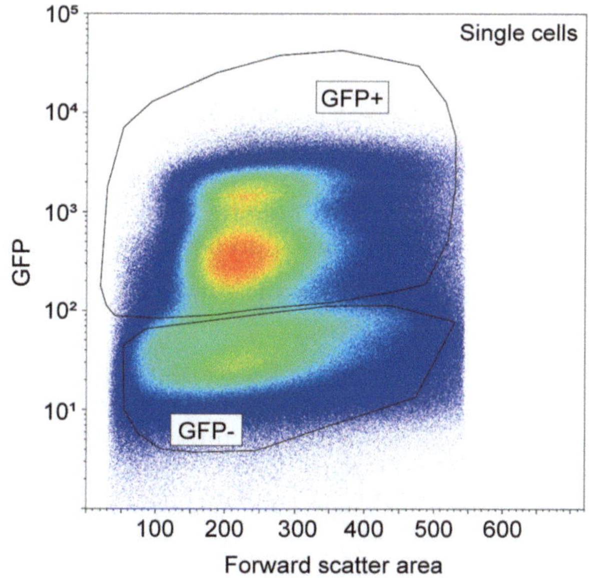

Fig. 1 Flow cytometry profile of formaldehyde-fixed cells dissociated from the MOEs of adult OMP-GFP+ mice. The forward scatter versus GFP signal is shown for single cell, after gating to remove doublets. The indicated gates were used to purify GFP+ cells for subsequent ChIP experiments

13. Pellet the sorted cells by centrifuging at 800 g for 10 min at 4 °C in a swinging bucket rotor. Carefully aspirate the supernatant. Flash freeze the cell pellet with liquid nitrogen and store at −80 °C, or proceed immediately to cell lysis and sonication.

3.2 Cell Lysis and Sonication

1. If cells were frozen, thaw the pellet gently on ice. Resuspend cell pellet in 1 mL lysis buffer, and transfer to a 1.5 mL microcentrifuge tube.
2. Incubate the cells in lysis buffer on ice for 10 min, and then pellet nuclei by centrifuging at 1000 g for 5 min at 4 °C.
3. Remove and discard the supernatant. Add 130 uL of shearing buffer, and gently resuspend the nuclei pellet by pipetting.
4. Transfer the resuspended nuclei to an AFA shearing vial and shear on a Covaris S220 ultrasonicator (*see* **Note 12**).
5. After shearing, transfer sonicated chromatin to a DNA LoBind 1.5 mL tube. Centrifuge at 10,000 g for 10 min at 4 °C to pellet insoluble material.
6. Transfer supernatant, which is the sonicated chromatin, to a new DNA LoBind 1.5 mL tube. At this point, small portions of the sonicated chromatin should be used for quantitative and qualitative analyses (*see* **Note 13**). Flash freeze the remaining chromatin in liquid nitrogen and store at −80 °C, or use immediately for chromatin immunoprecipitation.

3.3 Chromatin Immunoprecipitation

Perform all steps on ice or in a cold room unless otherwise noted. Use Eppendorf 1.5 mL LoBind microcentrifuge tubes throughout this portion of the protocol. All buffers must be prepared using nuclease-free water and pre-chilled to 4 °C. Include 1× Protease Inhibitor Cocktail, as indicated. Protease inhibitors are not required for the wash and elution steps. Pipet carefully throughout, avoiding bubbles. Work quickly when changing solutions on magnetic beads; do not allow the beads to dry.

1. **[Day 1]** If the sonicated chromatin was frozen, thaw gently on ice.
2. While the chromatin thaws, prepare Protein G Dynabeads. Resuspend the beads thoroughly by vortexing until no clumps persist, then transfer 44 uL, per IP, to a new 1.5 mL tube (*see* **Note 14**).
3. Pull down beads by placing the 1.5 mL tube on a magnetic rack until the solution clears, approximately 2 min, then remove the supernatant, and resuspend the beads in 1 mL of ChIP Dilution Buffer (CDB) by vortexing.
4. Repeat wash as in step 3.
5. Pull down the beads on magnet and remove the supernatant. Resuspend the beads in 44 uL (per IP) of CDB by pipetting.
6. Transfer half of the beads (22uL per IP) to a new 1.5 mL tube. These are the "Block" beads, which will be blocked overnight with yeast tRNA and then used for the IP on day 2. The remaining beads are the "Pre-clear" beads, which will be used to pre-clear any chromatin fragments that bind nonspecifically to beads before adding antibody.
7. To the "Block" beads, add CDB up to a total volume of 900 uL. Add 100 uL yeast tRNA (20 mg/mL) and then rotate *overnight at 4 °C*.
8. Once chromatin is thawed, setup a "pre-clear" tube for each IP reaction that will be performed. First, transfer 2–4 ug of chromatin to a new LoBind 1.5 mL tube (*see* **Note 15**). Then bring the volume up to 480 uL by adding CDB (with Protease Inhibitor Cocktail). Finally, add 20 uL of the reserved pre-clear beads. Rotate for 1 hour at 4 °C.
9. Pull down the beads by placing the tube on a magnet for 2 min. Transfer the supernatant, which is the pre-cleared chromatin, to a new tube. Discard the beads.
10. Transfer 10 uL of the pre-cleared chromatin, which constitutes a 2% input control, to a new tube. Place this "2% input control" tube at 4 °C until day 3.

11. Add 1 uL of anti-CTCF antibody to the cleared chromatin (*see* **Note 16**). Rotate the antibody and pre-cleared chromatin mixture *overnight at 4* °C.
12. **[Day 2]** Pull down the "Block" beads on the magnet, and discard the supernatant. Wash beads by adding 1 mL CDB and resuspend by pipetting.
13. Pull down the beads, and then discard the CDB wash. Add 110 uL CDB (per IP) and then resuspend by pipetting.
14. For each IP, transfer 100 uL of the washed and blocked bead solution to a new DNA LoBind tube. Discard any leftover beads.
15. Pull down the beads. Discard the CDB supernatant, and then immediately add ~500 uL antibody bound chromatin.
16. Rotate the beads together with antibody bound chromatin for 1 hour at 4 °C.
17. Pull down the beads. Discard the supernatant, and then add 1 mL LiCl wash buffer. Resuspend the beads by rotating for 3 min on rotary mixer in a 4 °C cold room.
18. Transfer the bead solution to a new LoBind tube (*see* **Note 17**).
19. Pull down beads and discard the supernatant. Add 1 mL LiCl wash buffer, then rotate for 3 min at 4 °C.
20. Repeat this wash three more times, for a total of four washes after transferring the beads to a new tube.
21. Pull down the beads and discard the supernatant. Add 1 mL of TE pH 7.5, then rotate for 3 min at 4 °C.
22. Pull down the beads and discard the supernatant. Add 100 uL of room temperature elution buffer with freshly added DTT, then resuspend by vortexing.
23. Incubate in a thermomixer at 65 °C with 900 rpm shaking for 30 min (*see* **Note 3**).
24. Pull down beads on magnet. Transfer supernatant (containing ChIP DNA), to a new LoBind tube.
25. Repeat elution with an additional 100 uL elution buffer + DTT. Pull down the beads and combine the second elution with the first (final volume 200 ul).
26. Dilute input control samples set aside on Day 1 by adding 190 uL of elution buffer + DTT, for a final volume of 200 uL.
27. Add 1 uL proteinase K (20 mg/mL) to each sample and input control. Pipet to mix.
28. Incubate *overnight at 65* °*C* in a heat block with a heated lid to reverse formaldehyde cross-links (*see* **Note 18**).

29. **[Day 3]** Column purify the eluted DNA and input control samples with a Zymo ChIP DNA Clean & Concentrator kit, or similar. First, dilute the samples using 1000 uL of binding buffer (5 volumes), then load this 1200 uL volume onto a single purification column in two 600 uL batches. Wash the column, and then elute twice with 10 uL of 10 mM Tris–HCl pH 8.0, collecting both eluates in the same DNA LoBind tube (final volume 20 ul).
30. Store ChIP DNA at −20 °C. Purified ChIP DNA can be analyzed by qPCR (Fig. 3; *see* **Note 19**) or used to prepare ChIP-seq libraries (*see* **Note 20**).

4 Notes

1. We recommend preparing 1% formaldehyde by diluting a freshly opened ampule of 16% methanol-free formaldehyde (e.g., Pierce #28906). Alternatively, a 1% formaldehyde solution can be prepared by heating paraformaldehyde, but care is required to avoid batch to batch variability in the efficiency of this process, which can lead to variable fixation efficiency.
2. Obtaining efficient and reproducible shearing of olfactory sensory neuron chromatin is challenging, perhaps due to the assembly of large heterochromatic foci. In our experience, Covaris focused ultrasonicators, such as the S2 or S220, greatly outperform other systems for this application. Covaris systems are able to shear olfactory sensory neuron chromatin to the ideal fragment size (200–300 bp) without heating the sample and are very consistent batch to batch.
3. If a shaking heat block is not available, vortex the samples every 5 min during the elution steps to keep Dynabeads in solution.
4. One vial of papain is sufficient to dissociate up to 10 adult MOEs. Use additional vials for larger-scale experiments.
5. Here we describe the purification of olfactory sensory neurons (OSNs) from mice bearing an OMP-GFP knock-in allele that specifically labels OSNs, but the same protocol can be applied with other labels and cell types, for example, OSNs labeled with OMP-Cre and Ai14 or INP3 cells labeled with an Ngn1-GFP BAC transgene.
6. One adult MOE will yield approximately one million OMP-GFP+ olfactory sensory neurons following papain dissociation and fluorescence-activated cell sorting. Thus, the recommended five mice should yield ~five million cells, which is a suitable number for sonication in a single shearing vial. This number can be scaled up or down as needed. Yields of OMP-GFP+ cells from newborn and juvenile animals increase with age. For example, at 2 weeks of age, each MOE will yield approximately 200,000 OMP-GFP+ OSNs.

7. For smaller-scale experiments using MOE tissue from juvenile mice or from only one to two adults, digest tissue with 1 mL papain in a 2 mL microcentrifuge tube. Perform the subsequent centrifugation steps in a 1.5 mL tube using a microcentrifuge tube swinging bucket adapter. Use a 1000 uL pipette with a trimmed tip to perform trituration steps. Prior to sorting, filter cells with a 40 um Flowmi cell strainer fitted to a 1000 uL pipet tip.
8. The optimal cross-linking time may vary depending on cell type and target protein. Additionally, alternative fixatives that form longer range cross-links, such as EGS (ethylene glycol bis(succinimidyl succinate)), may facilitate the capture of proteins that interact indirectly with DNA.
9. After fixation, all steps are performed at 4 °C or on ice.
10. The final dilution of dissociated cells may need to be adjusted depending on the needs of your flow cytometry instrument. Generally, a minimum volume of 500–600 uL is required. Beyond this minimum, we prefer to keep cells at a high concentration to facilitate rapid sorting of large numbers of cells. Even at high concentrations of cells, we observe very little clumping after the 40 um filtration step.
11. The specific parameters for sorting and collecting cells vary between instruments, but we have successfully sorted fixed OMP-GFP+ cells using a variety of instruments including the BD FACSAria II, the BD Influx, and the MoFlo Astrios EQ Cell Sorter. The brightness of the GFP reporter is reduced by formaldehyde fixation, but sufficient GFP signal should remain to identify and purify GFP+ cells (Fig. 1). During initial experiments, control mice that do not express GFP should be prepared in parallel to allow suitable gates to be configured. Alternatively, the sorting step can be skipped entirely, and the heterogeneous cell suspension can be lysed and sonicated for whole tissue cross-linked ChIP.
12. Sonication conditions should be optimized prior to starting immunoprecipitations, as the conditions required for shearing chromatin to the optimal fragment size (~200–300 bp) vary with cell type. For OSNs, we sonicate on a Covaris S220 ultrasonicator using the following settings: *duty cycle = 2%*, *peak power = 105 W*, *cycles per burst = 200*, *max temperature = 6 °C*, and *sonication time = 14 min*. It is generally possible to optimize shearing by varying the sonication time without changing other parameters. As a first step, we recommend testing a series of sonication times and then evaluating the distribution of sheared DNA products running 200–500 ng of purified DNA on an agarose gel (Fig. 2). For particularly challenging samples, it may be necessary to increase the concentration of SDS in the shearing buffer. Once optimal

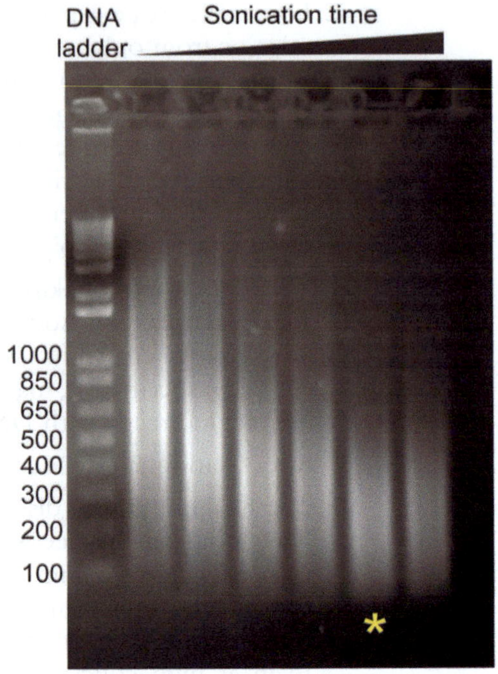

Fig. 2 Sonicated chromatin resolved on an agarose gel and stained with ethidium bromide. Increased sonication time results in a shift toward smaller fragment sizes. The lane marked with an asterisk has optimal shearing

conditions have been identified, ultrasonication is generally very consistent from batch to batch, Moreover, we have observed that shearing is generally not affected by cell number, with experiments ranging from 0.5 million to ten million cells per vial yielding very similar shearing. Nonetheless, the size distribution of the sonicated DNA should be checked for each batch of chromatin.

13. *To quantify the concentration of DNA in chromatin*, use a fluorescence-based assay for dsDNA, such as the PicoGreen or QuantiFluor. Depending on the assay, analyze 0.5–2 uL of chromatin per reaction. For five million cells sheared in a 130 uL vial, expect a concentration of ~100 ng/uL chromatin. *To analyze the distribution of product sizes of generated by sonication*, transfer 5–10 uL of chromatin to a PCR tube, and then bring the volume up to 25 uL with water. Add 1 uL RNase A (10 mg/mL), mix by pipetting, and then incubate for 30 min at 37 °C. Then add 1 uL Proteinase K (20 mg/mL), and incubate overnight at 65 °C. The next day, dilute each sample to 100 uL with water, then column purify the DNA with a Zymo DNA Clean & Concentrator kit or similar, eluting with 8 uL of elution buffer. Run the purified DNA on 1.5% agarose gel to check shearing (Fig. 2).

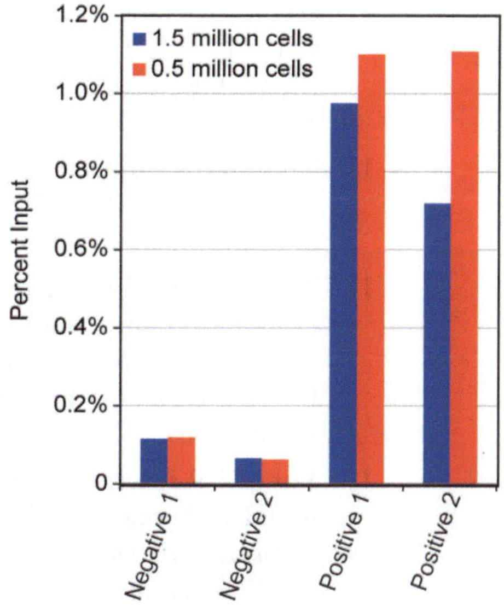

Fig. 3 Quantitative PCR analysis of a CTCF ChIP from 1.5 million and 0.5 million OMP-GFP+ OSNs for two CTCF binding sites and two negative control sites

14. Volumes in this and future steps are given as "per IP" in order to accommodate setting up multiple ChIP reactions in parallel. For example, if four different IPs will be setup in parallel, then use 176 uL of Protein G Dynabeads (4 x 44 uL) for step 2.

15. The amount of chromatin needed for a successful IP is antigen- and antibody-specific. We recommend 2–4 ug of chromatin per IP as a starting point. Addition of more chromatin is generally beneficial as it will result in recovering a greater quantity of DNA even if the IP efficiency is unchanged. However, it is also crucial to limit the total *volume* of sonicated chromatin that is added to the IP. This is because the shearing buffer contains 0.5% SDS, which can interfere with antibody binding. We recommend a maximum of 50 uL of chromatin per IP, yielding a final concentration of 0.05% SDS in the antibody binding reaction. This concentration of SDS is tolerated by many antibodies including CTCF. However, some antibodies may require further reducing this amount. If necessary, 10–20 million cells can be sheared together in the same shearing vial, increasing the concentration of the sonicated chromatin and thereby allowing a smaller *volume* of chromatin to be added to each IP. Finally, for quantitative experiments comparing IP efficiency between different conditions, the final concentration of SDS should be the same in each IP. This can be accomplished by adding additional shearing buffer to the more concentrated chromatin samples.

16. The quantity of antibody required for a successful IP varies. Considerations include the grade of the antibody and the

abundance and occupancy of the antigen. We recommend starting with 1 ug of antibody for 2–4ug of chromatin. For the CTCF polyclonal antibody used here, which is provided as antiserum, 1 uL is suitable.

17. This step eliminates any chromatin fragments that may have adhered nonspecifically to the plastic of the tube during the immunoprecipitation steps.
18. The heated lid prevents the 200 uL volume from completely evaporating and condensing at the top of the 1.5 mL tube. If not available, perform the overnight reverse crosslinking in a 0.5 mL DNA Lo-Bind tube, which limits evaporation, or use mineral oil.
19. For qPCR reactions, use 0.2 uL of ChIP or input DNA per well in a 10 uL reaction. Perform all qPCR reactions in technical triplicate. In order to calculate percent input, compare the ChIP signal in the ChIP DNA wells to the corresponding 2% input wells. We have utilized CTCF qPCR for positive and negative control sites for mouse OSNs.
20. The quantity of ChIP DNA recovered may be very small, depending on the identity of the target protein and antibody used, and the concentration after elution is frequently too low to quantify. We recommend using ultralow input kits for preparing ChIP-seq libraries, such as the Ovation Ultralow V2 system. We also recommend using a PCR-based library quantification assay, such as KAPA or Collibri, to measure the concentration of the ChIP DNA after the End Repair and Adapter Ligation steps of library preparation. This concentration can then be used to estimate the number of cycles of PCR required for library amplification.

References

1. Gilmour DS, Lis JT (1985) In vivo interactions of RNA polymerase II with genes of Drosophila melanogaster. Mol Cell Biol 5:2009–2018
2. Solomon MJ, Varshavsky A (1985) Formaldehyde-mediated DNA-protein crosslinking: a probe for in vivo chromatin structures. Proc Natl Acad Sci U S A 82:6470–6474
3. Hoffman EA, Frey BL, Smith LM et al (2015) Formaldehyde crosslinking: a tool for the study of chromatin complexes. J Biol Chem 290: 26404–26411
4. Johnson DS, Mortazavi A, Myers RM et al (2007) Genome-wide mapping of in vivo protein-DNA interactions. Science 316:1497–1502
5. Zhang Y, Liu T, Meyer CA et al (2008) Model-based Analysis of ChIP-Seq (MACS). Genome Biol 9:R137
6. Markenscoff-Papadimitriou E, Allen WE, Colquitt BM et al (2014) Enhancer interaction networks as a means for singular olfactory receptor expression. Cell 159:543–557
7. Monahan K, Schieren I, Cheung J et al (2017) Cooperative interactions enable singular olfactory receptor expression in mouse olfactory neurons. elife 6:1–32
8. Monahan K, Horta A, Lomvardas S (2019) LHX2- and LDB1-mediated trans interactions regulate olfactory receptor choice. Nature 565: 448–453
9. Shykind BM, Rohani SC, O'Donnell S et al (2004) Gene switching and the stability of odorant receptor gene choice. Cell 117:801–815

Chapter 7

Activity-Dependent Labeling of Olfactory Sensory Neurons Using RNA Fluorescence In Situ Hybridization Followed by Phospho-S6 Immunofluorescence

Maira Harume Nagai and Hiroaki Matsunami

Abstract

This microscope-based method allows demonstrating that an odorant receptor responded to an odorant in vivo. In sections of olfactory epithelium from odorant-exposed mice, the subpopulation of olfactory sensory neurons expressing a particular odorant receptor type is labeled using RNA fluorescence in situ hybridization. Sequential immunofluorescence against the phosphorylated S6 ribosomal subunit reveals the activated olfactory sensory neurons. The presence of double-labeled cells confirms that the particular odorant receptor type was activated by the odorant stimulation.

Key words Odorant stimulation, Odorant receptor (OR), Mature olfactory sensory neurons (mOSNS), RNA fluorescence in situ hybridization (RNA FISH), OR probe, Phosphorylated S6 (phospho-S6, pS6), Phospho-S6 immunofluorescence (pS6 IF)

1 Introduction

Odorant detection is initiated in the nasal cavity by the activation of odorant receptors (ORs) expressed in the cilia of mature olfactory sensory neurons (mOSNs) that compose the olfactory epithelium (OE). ORs belong to the largest subfamily of G-protein-coupled receptors (GPCRs) in the vertebrate genome and are encoded by over 1000 intact genes in mice [1–5]. Each odorant activates a specific subset of ORs, generating a combinatorial code of the odorant identity and increasing the discriminatory ability of the olfactory system [6–8]. The identification of odorant-OR interactions is essential to advance our understanding of the "olfactory code," and relies on data from in vitro, in vivo, and ex vivo approaches. The double-labeling of mOSNs using RNA fluorescence in situ hybridization (RNA FISH) and phospho-S6 immunofluorescence (pS6 IF) is instrumental in the validation of odorant-OR interactions in living animals (Fig. 1), as well as in the

Bradley J. Goldstein and Hiroaki Matsunami (eds.), *The Olfactory System*, Methods in Molecular Biology, vol. 2710,
https://doi.org/10.1007/978-1-0716-3425-7_7,

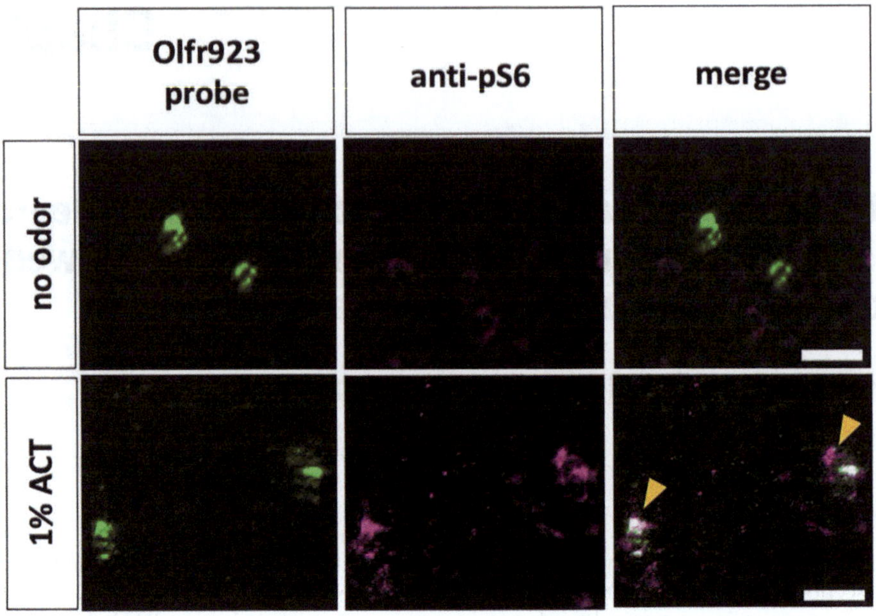

Fig. 1 Validation of OR response to odorant stimulation using RNA FISH and pS6 IF. mOSNs expressing Olfr923 were labeled by RNA FISH (green), and mOSNs activated by stimulation with 1% acetophenone (ACT) were labeled by pS6 IF (magenta). The presence of double-labeled cells (arrowheads) in odorant-exposed mice, but not in the control condition (no odor), confirms that odorant stimulation activated Olfr923-expressing mOSNs

quantitative analysis of OR activation across different stimulation conditions.

A single OR gene is predominantly expressed per mOSN, producing molecularly and functionally diverse subpopulations of mOSNs within the OE [6, 9–11]. RNA FISH is a powerful method that indicates the localization of a specific mRNA in fixed tissues, thus can be applied in OE sections to label mOSN subpopulations according to the expressed OR type. This method relies on the sequence-specific annealing property of nucleic acids and requires the sensitive hybridization of a known mRNA sequence to a labeled, complementary RNA probe. The mRNA: probe hybrids are detected using a fluorescent approach, finally revealing the mRNA location in the sample [12, 13]. Here we describe the OR probe preparation using a DNA plasmid as template, the tissue pretreatment to increase hybridization efficiency, the hybridization conditions, and the fluorescent detection of mRNA: OR probe hybrids using the tyramide signal amplification (TSA) system.

Active mOSNs are subsequently labeled through indirect immunofluorescence (IF) against the phosphorylated S6 ribosomal subunit (pS6). OE sections previously used in RNA FISH are incubated with an anti-pS6 primary antibody, followed by fluorophore-conjugated secondary antibody detection. In the brain, pS6 is a known readout of the neuronal response to multiple physiological and pharmacological stimuli and has been widely used as a marker of neuronal activity [14, 15]. pS6 was shown to be triggered in the mouse OE by odorant exposure and has been successfully used to track mOSN activation [16–18]. Since OR expression by mOSNs is monogenic, the double-labeling using RNA FISH and pS6 IF allows directly associating the odorant response with a particular OR type.

2 Materials

2.1 OE Sections

1. 3-week-old mouse.
2. Disposable animal container with lid.
3. Odorant of interest.
4. 1.5 cm × 1.5 cm pieces of blotting paper.
5. Plastic cassette with lid (e.g., Sakura Tissue-Tek® Uni-Cassette).
6. Histology mold.
7. OCT compound.
8. Adhesion glass slides, treated for use with frozen tissue sections.
9. Cryostat.

2.2 OR Probe Preparation

2.2.1 PCR Amplification of DNA Template

1. Plasmid DNA containing the OR sequence (1–10 ng/μL) (*see* **Note 1**).
2. Nuclease-free water.
3. 10× standard PCR buffer.
4. dNTP mix (2 mM each).
5. 5 μM forward primer (*see* **Note 1**).
6. 5 μM reverse primer (T3 RNA polymerase promoter sequenced added to the 5′ end) (*see* **Notes 1** and **2**).
7. Taq DNA polymerase (5 U/μl) (*see* **Note 3**).
8. PCR purification kit.
9. 1% agarose gel.
10. DNA molecular weight marker.
11. Thermocycler.

2.2.2 Riboprobe Synthesis

1. Purified DNA template (from Subheading 2.2.1).
2. Nuclease-free water.
3. 5× RNA polymerase buffer: 200 mM Tris–HCl (pH 7.9 at 25 °C), 30 mM $MgCl_2$, 10 mM spermidine, 50 mM NaCl (*see* **Note 2**).

4. 10× DIG RNA labeling mix: 10 mM ATP, CTP, GTP (each), 6.5 mM UTP, 3.5 mM DIG-11-UTP (*see* **Note 4**).
5. RNase inhibitor mix: 1:1 mix of RNase inhibitors [Qiagen #129916 or Ambion #AM2682, and RNasin Promega #N2511].
6. T3 RNA polymerase (10–20 U/μl) (*see* **Note 2**).
7. 100 mM DTT.
8. RNase-free 1 M $NaHCO_3$.
9. RNase-free 1 M Na_2CO_3.
10. RNAse-free riboprobe purification columns.
11. Deionized formamide.
12. Thermocyclers.

2.3 RNA FISH

Use RNase-free reagents, solutions, plasticware, and glassware in the pre-hybridization and hybridization steps.

2.3.1 Pre-hybridization and Hybridization

1. Slides containing 18–20 μm OE cryosections.
2. Deionized water (dH_2O).
3. 1× PBS.
4. Acetic anhydride.
5. Triethanolamine solution (prepare immediately before use): in a 1 L glass beaker, mix 8.2 mL of triethanolamine and 800 mL of dH_2O using a magnetic stirrer.
6. Pre-hybridization buffer (stored at −20 °C): 50% (v/v) formamide, 5× SSC buffer, 250 μg/mL baker's yeast RNA, 100 μg/mL herring or salmon sperm DNA, 1 mM DTT, 300 U/mL heparin, adjust volume with nuclease-free water.
7. Fresh 4% formaldehyde solution (prepare on the day of the experiment): in the chemical hood, mix 1.6 g of paraformaldehyde (PFA), 1 mL of 10 N NaOH, and 300 mL of dH_2O using a magnetic stirrer. When PFA is dissolved (~1 h), add 17 mL of 20× RNase-free PBS, and adjust pH to 7–8 with 10 N HCl (~900 μL). Complete the volume to 400 mL with dH_2O and vacuum filter to remove undissolved particles. PFA is toxic; keep the solution covered and avoid inhalation.
8. Soaking buffer (store at 4 °C): 50% formamide, 5× SSC buffer, adjust volume with dH_2O.
9. OR probe (from Subheading 2.2) .
10. Parafilm.
11. Staining buckets.
12. Slide rack with handle.

13. Slide holders (made with Petri dish and 1 mL serological pipettes) (*see* **Note 5**).
14. Blotting paper.
15. Paper towels.
16. Magnetic stirrer and magnetic bar.
17. 2 mL or 5 mL serological pipette.
18. Plastic containers.
19. Laboratory oven.

2.3.2 Post-hybridization Washes and Fluorescent Detection Using TSA

1. 1× PBS.
2. 0.2× SSC buffer.
3. 5× SSC buffer.
4. 5% stock blocking solution: dissolve 10 g of Blocking Reagent [Roche #11096176001] in 200 mL of maleic acid buffer. Autoclave and store at 4 °C.
5. 7.5% BSA solution [Gibco #A8412].
6. 30% H_2O_2.
7. Tyramide-fluorescein stock (light-sensitive, must be protected from light): prepare 10 mg/mL NHS-fluorescein solution (40 mg NHS-fluorescein, 4 mL dimethylformamide) and 10 mg/mL tyramide solution (20 mg tyramide, 2 mL dimethylformamide, 20 μL triethylamine). Mix 4 mL of NHS-fluorescein solution and 1.37 mL tyramide solution, and incubate at room temperature for 2 h. Add 4.6 mL of ethanol and store at −20 °C.
8. Antibody anti-DIG-POD (*see* **Note 6**).
9. Parafilm.
10. Staining buckets.
11. Slide mailers.
12. Coplin jars.
13. Slide rack with handle.
14. Slide holders (as in Subheading 2.3.1).
15. Tweezers.
16. Paper towels.
17. Water bath.

2.4 pS6 IF

1. 1× PBS.
2. dH_2O.
3. Skim milk powder.
4. PBST: 0.1% Triton X-100, 1× PBS.

5. Primary antibody (anti-phospho-S6 (Ser240/244) (D68F8) [Cell Signaling #5364]).
6. Secondary antibody (Cy3-conjugate anti-rabbit IgG [Jackson Immuno Research #711-165-152]).
7. Nuclei stain solution.
8. Slide mailers.
9. Staining buckets.
10. Mounting medium.
11. Glass coverslips.

3 Methods

3.1 OE Sections (Fig. 2)

1. In a fume hood (environment free of contaminant odorants), habituate a 3-week-old mouse for 1 h inside a disposable container tightly closed.
2. Pipette 10 μL of odorant (diluted or undiluted) onto a piece of blotting paper. For control animals, use 10 μL of solvent (typically water or ethanol). Enclose the blotting paper in the plastic cassette, and place it in a second container.
3. Transfer the habituated mouse to the second container and close it tightly. After 1 h, euthanize the mouse using CO_2.
4. Decapitate the mouse. Dissect the nose, removing the skin, lower mandible with tongue, palate, and teeth.
5. Embed the dissected nose in the histology mold with OCT compound. Freeze in dry ice/ethanol bath and store at −80 °C.
6. Section the nose tissue using a cryostat. Collect 18–20 μm sections on adhesion slides. Store slides at −80 °C.

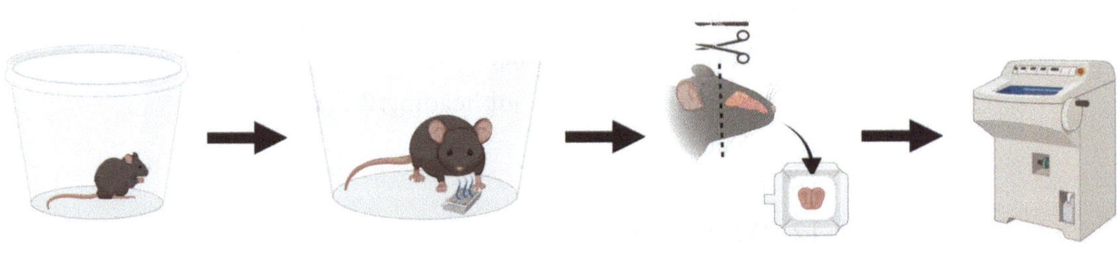

Fig. 2 Outline of the main steps to prepare OE sections from odorant-stimulated mice. The animal is habituated in a disposable container (e.g., paper bucket with lid) and then transferred to a second container containing the odorant source. After exposure to the odorant, the mouse is euthanized. The animal's nose is dissected and frozen in OCT. The tissue is sectioned using a cryostat. If preparing control mice, expose the mice to solvent instead of odorant. (Created with BioRender.com)

Table 1
PCR reaction mix to amplify probe template DNA

Reagent	Volume (μL)	Final concentration
Plasmid DNA (1–10 ng/μL)	1	0.1–1 ng/μL
10× standard PCR buffer	1	1×
2 mM dNTPs (each)	1	0.2 mM (each)
5 μM forward primer	1	0.5 μM
5 μM reverse primer	1	0.5 μM
Taq DNA polymerase (5 U/μL) (see Note 2)	0.05	0.025 U/μL
Nuclease-free water	5	
Total	10	

Table 2
PCR cycling conditions to amplify probe template DNA

Step	Temperature	Time
Initial denaturation	95 °C	15 min
25 cycles	95 °C Variable (adjust to primer sequence) 72 °C	15 sec 15 sec Variable (1 min/template bp kb)
Final extension	72 °C	5 min

3.2 OR Probe Preparation

3.2.1 PCR Amplification of DNA Template

1. Set up the PCR reaction (Table 1), and run it for 25 PCR cycles (Table 2) (*see* **Note 3**).
2. Clean up the amplified DNA template using the PCR purification kit. We use the MinElute PCR purification kit [Qiagen #28004], which allows a final elution in a small volume (10 μL) of EB buffer (10 mM Tris–HCl, pH 8.5). We follow the supplier's instructions, which are briefly described below (all centrifugations are performed at maximum speed):
   2.1. Add 200 μL of PB buffer to the PCR reaction and mix thoroughly.
   2.2. Transfer the mixture to the columns and centrifuge for 30 seconds.
   2.3. Wash the columns by adding 750 μL of PE buffer and centrifuging for 30 seconds.
   2.4. Discard the flow-through, and centrifuge for 2 min to remove the remaining PE buffer.

Table 3
Transcription reaction mix to synthesize RNA probe

Reagent	20 μL reaction	10 μL reaction (half-sized)
Purified template DNA	2 μL	1 μL
5× RNA polymerase buffer	4 μL	2 μL
DIG RNA labeling mix	2 μL	1 μL
RNase inhibitor mix	1 μL	0.5 μL
T3 RNA Pol	1 μL	0.5 μL
DTT (100 mM)	2 μL	1 μL
Nuclease-free water	8 μL	4 μL

2.5. Discard the collection tube and place the column into a clean microcentrifuge tube.

2.6. Add 10 μL of EB buffer to the center of the column and centrifuge for 2 min to elute the PCR product.

3. Run 1 μL of purified DNA template in 1% agarose gel electrophoresis to check for successful recovery of PCR product. A strong and sharp band (typically ~50–150 ng/μL) must be seen. If a faint or diffuse band is obtained, optimize the PCR reaction.

3.2.2 Probe Synthesis, Hydrolysis, and Cleanup

1. Set up the transcription reaction (Table 3), and incubate for 120 min at 37 °C (*see* **Note 2**). Hold at 4 °C if not proceed immediately to **step 3**.
2. Meanwhile, prepare the alkaline buffer (80 mM $NaHCO_3$, 120 mM Na_2CO_3): for 150 μL total, mix 12 μL of 1 M $NaHCO_3$, 18 μL of 1 M Na_2CO_3, and 120 μL of nuclease-free water. This volume is enough for three full-size or six half-size transcription reactions.
3. Hydrolyze the probe by adding 25 μL (for half-size) or 50 μL (for full-size) of alkaline buffer to the transcription reaction and incubating at 60 °C for 15 min.
4. Clean up the reaction using an RNase-free riboprobe purification column. We use the Micro Bio-Spin 30 columns [Bio-Rad #732-6223], following the supplier's instructions. The procedure is briefly described below:

4.1. Invert the column several times to resuspend the Bio-gel, and remove bubbles.

4.2. Snap off the column's bottom tip, and insert the column into a collection tube (included).

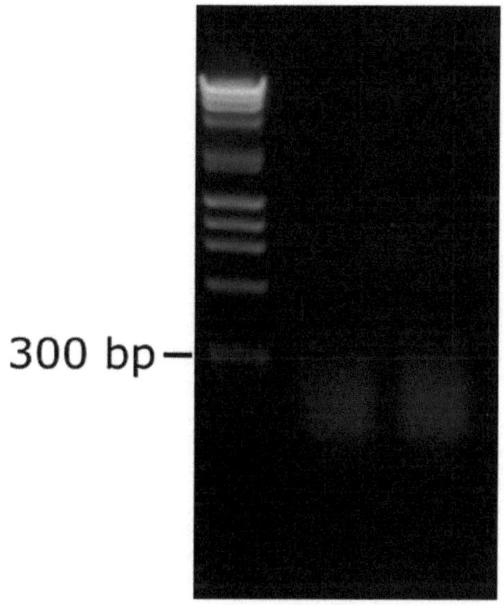

Fig. 3 Representative image of two OR probes after hydrolysis and purification. A smear between 100 and 200 bp DNA markers is observed

4.3. Remove the column's cap, and let the packing buffer flow by gravity until it is drained.

4.4. Discard the buffer e place the column back in the same tube.

4.5. Centrifuge the column at 1000× *g* for 2 min. Discard the collection tube and remaining packing buffer.

4.6. Insert the column in a clean microcentrifuge tube. Carefully pipette the probe on the top center of the column, and centrifuge at 1000× *g* for 4 min.

5. Add 1:1 volume of deionized formamide to the eluted probe (70 μL for full-size reaction, 35 μL for half-size).
6. Run 5 μL of riboprobe in 1% agarose gel electrophoresis. The product should correspond to a smear between 100 and 200 bp DNA markers (Fig. 3). Store probe at −80 °C.

3.3 RNA FISH

3.3.1 Pre-hybridization (Day 1)

Before starting, turn the oven on at 58 °C, and wipe the bench and pipettes with 70% ethanol. Prepare the slide holder by placing a blotting paper in the Petri dish, wetting the blotting paper with soaking buffer, and making two parallel rails with 1 mL serological pipettes. Snap the pipettes tips to fit the Petri dish (Fig. 4).

1. Take the slides from −80 °C, and place them on a flat, clean surface (e.g., a plastic tray cleaned with 70% ethanol). Using a hair dryer, blow the slides until the condensation droplets evaporate.

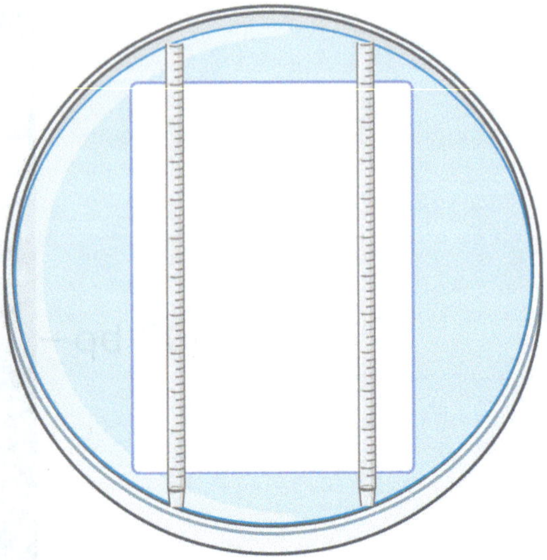

Fig. 4 Slide holders made with a 150 mm diameter Petri dish and 1 mL serological pipettes. For overnight incubation of slides, place a blotting paper wet with soaking buffer (RNA FISH) or a paper towel wet with dH_2O (pS6 IF) on the bottom of the Petri dish. (Created with BioRender.com)

2. Label the slides using a pencil or waterproof marker, and load them on a slide rack.
3. Dip the slide rack in a staining bucket containing 4% formaldehyde. Incubate for 15 min.
4. Transfer the slide rack to a new bucket containing 1× PBS, and incubate for 5 min.
5. Repeat **step 4**.
6. Gently stir the triethanolamine solution in the glass beaker using a magnetic stirrer. Dip in the slide rack until the slides are fully immersed, using a serological pipette to hold the slide rack away from the beaker's bottom (Fig. 5).
7. Add 1.75 mL of acetic anhydride to the triethanolamine solution, and incubate the slides for 10 min. The acetic anhydride must be added dropwise within the first minute of incubation.
8. Transfer the slide rack to a new bucket containing 1× PBS and incubate for 5 min.
9. Take one slide at a time, remove excess fluid onto paper towels, and dry the back and laterals of the slide using blotting paper. Place the slide on the rails of the slide holder, and pipette 500 μL of pre-hybridization buffer onto the tissue sections. After all the slides are done, incubate the slide holder in the oven at 58 °C for at least 1 h.

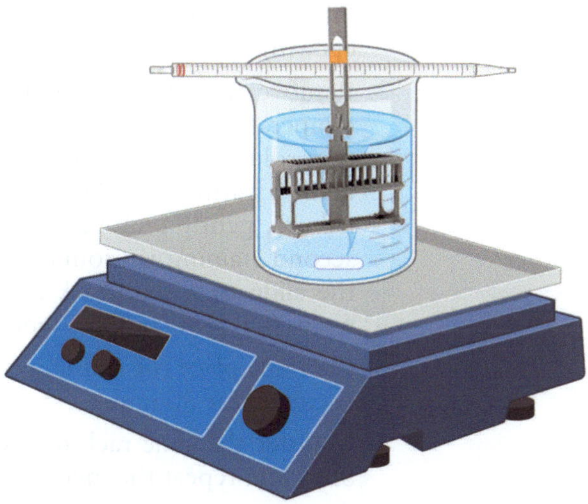

Fig. 5 Tissue treatment with triethanolamine + acetic anhydride during pre-hybridization. The slide rack must be fully immersed in the solution without touching the bottom of the beaker. Use a serological pipette to suspend the slide rack. Keep the solution under gentle stirring using a magnetic stirrer. (Created with BioRender.com)

3.3.2 Hybridization (Day 1)

Before starting, line a plastic container with blotting paper, and wet the blotting paper with soaking buffer. The plastic container must be large enough to fit the slide holders.

1. Prepare the hybridization solution (200 μl per slide): for 200 μl of pre-hybridization buffer, we typically use 1 μl of diluted (1: 100–1:10) probe when the OR CDS was used as template, or 1–3 μl of undiluted probe when the OR UTR was used as template. The best probe concentration must be experimentally determined (*see* **Note** 7).
2. Heat the hybridization solution at 85 °C for 5 min.
3. Move the slides to room temperature.
4. Take one slide at a time from the slide holder. Remove pre-hybridization buffer onto paper towels, and dry the back and laterals of the slide using blotting paper. Place the slide on the slide holder and add hybridization solution. Cover the slide with a slide-wide strip of parafilm to form a coverslip. After all the slides are done, place the slide holders in the plastic container. Incubate overnight at 58 °C.

3.3.3 Post-Hybridization Washes and Fluorescent Detection Using TSA (Day 2)

Before starting, warm the 0.5× SSC and 5× SSC buffers to 72 °C in a water bath. In the meantime, make 0.5% blocking solution (dilute 5% stock blocking solution in 1× PBS) and 0.1% BSA solution (dilute 7.5% BSA in 1× PBS).

1. Fill two Coplin jars with warm 5× SSC and two staining buckets with warm 0.2× SSC.
2. Remove the slides from the oven and place them at room temperature. Take one slide at a time, remove excess hybridization solution onto paper towels, and dip in a Coplin jar containing warm 5× SSC buffer. If the parafilm coverslip does not fall off, gently remove it with tweezers. Rinse the slide in a second staining jar containing warm 5× SSC buffer. Transfer the slide to a slide rack inside a staining bucket containing warm 0.2× SSC buffer. Repeat until all slides are done.
3. Carefully place the staining bucket in the water bath at 72 °C. Incubate for 30 min.
4. Transfer the slide rack to a second jar containing warm 0.2× SSC, and repeat the incubation in the water bath.
5. Transfer the slide rack to a staining jar containing 1× PBS, and incubate for 5 min at room temperature.
6. Load slides in a slide mailer containing 0.5% blocking buffer, and incubate for 30 min. In the last 5 min of incubation, prepare antibody solution by diluting 1:1000 anti-DIG-POD in the 0.5% blocking buffer.
7. Take one slide at a time from the mailer. Use paper towels to remove excess fluid and dry the back and laterals of the slide. Place the slide on the slide holder, and add 300 μl of antibody solution per slide. After all the slides are done, incubate for 45 min.
8. Discard the antibody solution onto paper towels, and place slides in the mailer. Rinse slides twice with 1× PBS (*see* **Note 8**).
9. Wash three times with 1× PBS for 10 min.
10. Replace 1× PBS with 0.1% BSA solution.
11. Prepare the TSA working solution (300 μl per slide): make 0.003% H_2O_2 (1:1000 dilution of 30% H_2O_2 in 1× PBS), then add 1:400 tyramide-fluorescein stock.
12. From this step on, the slides must be protected from light. Take one slide at a time from the slide mailer; use paper towels to remove excess fluid, and dry the back and laterals of the slide. Place the slide on the slide holder, and add 300 μl of TSA working solution per slide. Incubate for 10 min.
13. Remove the TSA working solution onto paper towels, and place the slides in the mailer. Rinse the slides twice with 1× PBS.
14. Wash with 1× PBS for at least 5 min.

3.4 pS6 IF (Days 2 and 3)

Before starting, prepare milk blocking by dissolving 5% (w/v) skim milk powder in PBST. Make slide holders by lining the Petri dish with a paper towel wet with dH_2O and using 1 mL serological pipettes as rails (Fig. 4).

1. Replace 1× PBS in the slide mailers with milk blocking and incubate for 30 min. In the last 5 min of incubation, prepare primary antibody solution by diluting 1:300 primary antibody in milk blocking.
2. Take one slide at a time from the slide mailer. Use paper towels to remove excess fluid, and dry the back and laterals of the slide. Place the slide on the slide holder, and add 300 μl of primary antibody solution per slide. Cover with a slide-wide strip of parafilm to form a coverslip. After all the slides are done, incubate overnight at 4 °C.
3. Move the slide tray to room temperature. Take one slide at a time, remove excess liquid onto paper towels, and place it in a slide mailer. Rinse the slides twice with 1× PBS.
4. Wash the slides three times with 1× PBS for at least 5 min each wash.
5. During the last wash, prepare secondary antibody solution by diluting 1:200 secondary antibody in milk blocking.
6. Take one slide at a time from the slide mailer. Use paper towels to remove excess fluid and dry the back and laterals of the slide. Place the slide on the slide holder, and add 300 μl of secondary antibody solution per slide. After all the slides are done, incubate for 45 min.
7. Remove secondary antibody solution onto paper towels, and place the slides in a mailer. Rinse slides twice with 1× PBS.
8. Replace 1× PBS in the slide mailers with nuclei staining solution and incubate for 5 min.
9. Discard the nuclei staining solution, and wash the slides twice with 1× PBS, incubating for at least 5 min each time.
10. Replace 1× PBS with dH_2O. Take one slide at a time from the mailer, remove excess liquid onto paper towels, and close it with mounting medium and coverslip.

4 Notes

1. The complete OR coding sequence (~1000 bp) can be used as template to synthesize the OR riboprobe. However, due to the high nucleotide identity shared by members of the same OR subfamily, stretches of the OR coding sequence (CDS) or untranslated regions (UTR) with low similarity to other ORs

can be used instead. We have successfully used as template UTR stretches as small as ~300 bp. The OR template is cloned into a vector of choice, and the PCR primers must flank the insert. The reverse primer is designed to contain an RNA polymerase promoter sequence in the 5′ end, which matches the RNA polymerase used to synthesize the complementary (antisense) OR riboprobe. A control (sense) riboprobe, which should yield no RNA FISH signal, can be synthesized if the RNA polymerase promoter is added to the forward PCR primer instead.

2. We routinely use T3 RNA polymerase (10–20 U/μl) [Promega #P2083] to synthesize the antisense OR probe, therefore the reactions are described for this reagent. If using a different enzyme or supplier, adjust the transcription reaction accordingly (e.g., enzyme volume and incubation temperature).
3. We use HotStarTaq DNA polymerase (5 U/μL) [Qiagen #203203], therefore the PCR reaction and cycling conditions are described for this reagent. If using a different enzyme or supplier, adjust the reaction accordingly (e.g., Taq volume, denaturation and polymerization conditions).
4. Alternatively, a 10× Fluorescein RNA labeling mix (10 mM ATP, 10 mM CTP, 10 mM GTP, 6.5 mM UTP, 3.5 mM Fluorescein-12-UTP) can be used.
5. A slide staining rack with paper towels saturated with soaking buffer can also be used.
6. If using fluorescein-labeled riboprobes, use anti-fluorescein-POD antibody.
7. This concentration range is used for DIG-labeled OR riboprobes. For fluorescein-labeled riboprobes, quantities can be 4× higher.
8. Carefully replace the solution in the slide mailers by holding the slides in place with a finger, and gently pouring off the solution. Pipette or pour the clean solution into the mailer avoiding direct flush onto the slides.

References

1. Buck L, Axel R (1991) A novel multigene family may encode odorant receptors: a molecular basis for odor recognition. Cell 65(1):175–187
2. Zhang X, Firestein S (2002) The olfactory receptor gene superfamily of the mouse. Nat Neurosci 5(2):124–133. https://doi.org/10.1038/nn800
3. Godfrey PA, Malnic B, Buck LB (2004) The mouse olfactory receptor gene family. Proc Natl Acad Sci U S A 101(7):2156–2161. https://doi.org/10.1073/pnas.0308051100
4. Barnes IHA, Ibarra-Soria X, Fitzgerald S, Gonzalez JM, Davidson C, Hardy MP, Manthravadi D, Van Gerven L, Jorissen M, Zeng Z, Khan M, Mombaerts P, Harrow J, Logan DW, Frankish A (2020) Expert curation of the human and mouse olfactory receptor gene repertoires identifies conserved coding regions split across two exons. BMC Genomics 21(1):196. https://doi.org/10.1186/s12864-020-6583-3
5. Niimura Y, Matsui A, Touhara K (2014) Extreme expansion of the olfactory receptor

gene repertoire in African elephants and evolutionary dynamics of orthologous gene groups in 13 placental mammals. Genome Res 24(9): 1485–1496. https://doi.org/10.1101/gr.169532.113

6. Malnic B, Hirono J, Sato T, Buck LB (1999) Combinatorial receptor codes for odors. Cell 96(5):713–723
7. Bozza T, Feinstein P, Zheng C, Mombaerts P (2002) Odorant receptor expression defines functional units in the mouse olfactory system. J Neurosci 22(8):3033–3043. https://doi.org/10.1523/JNEUROSCI.22-08-03033.2002
8. Saito H, Chi Q, Zhuang H, Matsunami H, Mainland JD (2009) Odor coding by a mammalian receptor repertoire. Sci Signal 2(60): 1–14. https://doi.org/10.1126/scisignal.2000016
9. Chess A, Simon I, Cedar H, Axel R (1994) Allelic inactivation regulates olfactory receptor gene expression. Cell 78(5):823–834. https://doi.org/10.1016/s0092-8674(94)90562-2
10. Hanchate NK, Kondoh K, Lu Z, Kuang D, Ye X, Qiu X, Pachter L, Trapnell C, Buck LB (2015) Single-cell transcriptomics reveals receptor transformations during olfactory neurogenesis. Science 350(6265):1251–1255. https://doi.org/10.1126/science.aad2456
11. Saraiva LR, Ibarra-Soria X, Khan M, Omura M, Scialdone A, Mombaerts P, Marioni JC, Logan DW (2015) Hierarchical deconstruction of mouse olfactory sensory neurons: from whole mucosa to single-cell RNA-seq. Sci Rep 5: 18178. https://doi.org/10.1038/srep18178
12. Singer RH, Ward DC (1982) Actin gene expression visualized in chicken muscle tissue culture by using in situ hybridization with a biotinated nucleotide analog. Proc Natl Acad Sci U S A 79(23):7331–7335. https://doi.org/10.1073/pnas.79.23.7331
13. Young AP, Jackson DJ, Wyeth RC (2020) A technical review and guide to RNA fluorescence in situ hybridization. PeerJ 8:e8806. https://doi.org/10.7717/peerj.8806
14. Knight ZA, Tan K, Birsoy K, Schmidt S, Garrison JL, Wysocki RW, Emiliano A, Ekstrand MI, Friedman JM (2012) Molecular profiling of activated neurons by phosphorylated ribosome capture. Cell 151(5):1126–1137. https://doi.org/10.1016/j.cell.2012.10.039
15. Biever A, Valjent E, Puighermanal E (2015) Ribosomal Protein S6 Phosphorylation in the Nervous System: From Regulation to Function. Front Mol Neurosci 8:75. https://doi.org/10.3389/fnmol.2015.00075
16. Jiang Y, Gong NN, Hu XS, Ni MJ, Pasi R, Matsunami H (2015) Molecular profiling of activated olfactory neurons identifies odorant receptors for odors in vivo. Nat Neurosci 18(10):1446–1454. https://doi.org/10.1038/nn.4104
17. Hu XS, Ikegami K, Vihani A, Zhu KW, Zapata M, de March CA, Do M, Vaidya N, Kucera G, Bock C, Jiang Y, Yohda M, Matsunami H (2020) Concentration-dependent recruitment of mammalian odorant receptors. eNeuro 7(2). https://doi.org/10.1523/ENEURO.0103-19.2019
18. Vihani A, Hu XS, Gundala S, Koyama S, Block E, Matsunami H (2020) Semiochemical responsive olfactory sensory neurons are sexually dimorphic and plastic. eLife 9:1–61. https://doi.org/10.7554/eLife.54501

Chapter 8

Measuring Cell Surface Expression of Odorant Receptors via Flow Cytometry

Jeevan Tewari and Hiroaki Matsunami

Abstract

Odorant receptor proteins (ORs) have highly variable cell surface expression levels. The majority of both human and murine ORs depend on chaperone proteins to traffic from the endoplasmic reticulum to the cell surface, while a limited subset of ORs express at high levels independently. Quantifying these heterogeneous expression levels is of high import for understanding the trafficking and stability of these integral-transmembrane proteins and for normalizing in vitro activation assays. Recognizable epitopes like the rhodopsin-tag can be inserted upstream of the N-termini in ORs to enable cell surface immunostaining and detection via flow cytometry. This method enables robust measurement and comparison of cell surface expression levels of different ORs. Our approach also facilitates the study of different chaperone proteins' effects on OR trafficking and expression.

Key words Odorant receptor, Olfactory receptor, Cell surface expression, Flow cytometry, Immunostaining, Receptor trafficking, Integral membrane proteins

1 Introduction

Olfaction relies on the detection of volatile compounds via integral membrane proteins termed odorant receptors. These ORs belong to class A of the G-protein-coupled receptor family and constitute the largest subfamily within this class [1]. The nearly 400 functionally expressed human odorant receptors maintain heterogeneity in amino acid sequence, enabling humans to detect and discriminate between molecules within the vast odorant chemical space [2, 3]. Researchers theorize that the diversification of the OR subfamily exchanged structural stability of odorant receptors for the ability to sense a more diverse set of odorants [4]. Thus, the majority of odorant receptors express poorly outside of nonolfactory cells. In heterologous cell systems, ORs are typically retained within the endoplasmic reticulum, failing to fold and traffic to the plasma membrane in sufficient quantities to enable odor detection

Bradley J. Goldstein and Hiroaki Matsunami (eds.), *The Olfactory System*, Methods in Molecular Biology, vol. 2710,
https://doi.org/10.1007/978-1-0716-3425-7_8,

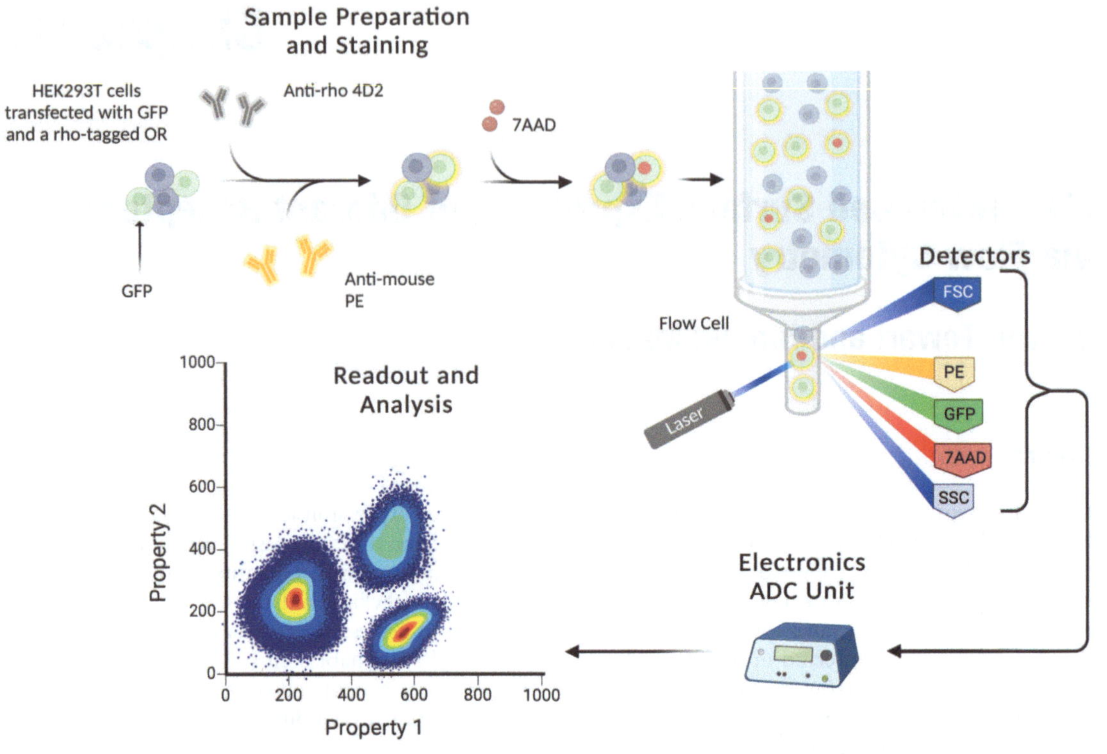

Fig. 1 Cartoon representation of flow cytometry. This diagram outlines the major components of a flow cytometry experimental pipeline from sample staining to analysis. Note that the forward scatter (FSC) detector receives spectral input from a path parallel to the excitatory laser. The side-scatter (SSC) and fluorescence detectors, represented by phycoerythrin (PE), green-fluorescent protein (GFP), and 7-aminoactinomycin-D (7AAD), receive input from light-scattered perpendicularly from cells. The analog-to-digital converter (ADC) unit is responsible for converting voltages resulting from spectral emission into digital information. In newer cytometers, this unit is found onboard the cytometers' electronics systems. Analysis and gating often involves selecting from a heterogeneous population of cells displayed on a dot plot based on select properties like FSC, SSC, or fluorescence

and membrane depolarization [4]. Olfactory sensory neurons overcome this issue of OR retention by expressing chaperone proteins like receptor transport proteins (RTPs) which facilitate OR folding and bolster cell surface expression [5]. Flow cytometry and cell surface immunostaining enables investigations into the magnitude of chaperone proteins' effects on expression and the detection of differences in receptor trafficking efficiency within the OR family.

Flow cytometry is a tool that integrates fluidics and optics to measure certain cell properties like light scattering or fluorescence. Broadly, this technique can be subdivided into three parts: the microfluidics system, the optics system, and the electronics as shown in Fig. 1. The fluidics system receives input from sample tubes containing suspended and fluorescently labeled cells. The microfluidics relies on hydrodynamic focusing, which utilizes a liquid flow sheath to generate an extremely narrow channel, wide enough for cells to move in a single file. The optics system contains an excitatory laser and two detector paths which are orthogonal to each other and the direction of the channel flow. These detectors enable measurement of cell properties like circularity, granularity, size, and a variety of fluorescence wavelength ranges.

This protocol contains all of the requisite steps to leverage flow cytometry for the determination of cell surface expression of ORs. We describe in detail five steps: plate seeding, transfection, sample staining, sample reading, and analysis. The user may customize this protocol by incorporating their own ORs of interest, different fluorescent components, and unique parameters in the analysis or flow cytometry software.

2 Materials

2.1 Equipment and Software

1. BD FACSCanto™ system with BD FACSDiva™ software.
2. Sterile culture fume hood and incubator.
3. Centrifuge that accommodates 5 mL polystyrene tubes.
4. Computer with FlowJo™ installed.

2.2 Reagents and Labware

1. 35/10 cm TC-treated cell culture dish with HEK293T cells grown to 100% confluence.
2. 6-well clear flat bottom TC-treated multiwell cell culture plates with lids.
3. 5 mL polystyrene round bottom tubes.
4. 50 mL conical centrifuge tubes.
5. 15 ml conical centrifuge tubes.
6. Cellstripper.
7. Phosphate buffered saline (PBS).
8. Minimal Essential Media (MEM).
9. M10: MEM containing 10% fetal bovine serum (FBS) and 1% mL GlutaMAX.
10. M10PSF: M10 containing 0.5% penicillin/streptomycin (10,000 units/ml and 10 mg/ml) and 1.25 ug/mL amphotericin B.
11. RTP1S: 100 ng/uL plasmid from H. Matsunami Lab.
12. Rho-tagged OR: 100 ng/uL plasmid (*see* **Note 1**).
13. GFP: 100 ng/uL plasmid.
14. Lipofectamine 2000 (1 mg/mL).
15. Mouse anti-rho4D2 antibody (50% glycerol v/v).

16. R-Phycoerythrin AffiniPure F(ab')$_2$ Fragment Donkey Anti-Mouse IgG (0.1 mg/ml) (Jackson Immunologicals: 715–116-150).
17. 7-Aminoactinomycin D (1 mg/mL).
18. Incubation solution: PBS containing 2% FBS and 15 mM sodium azide.

3 Methods

3.1 Plate Seeding

1. Remove the 100% confluence cell culture plate from the incubator, and vacuum the growth media.
2. Wash the plate by pipetting 10 mL PBS onto the side of the plate and vacuum the wash.
3. Pipette 3 mL of trypsin EDTA directly onto the plate and let plate incubate for 3–5 min.
4. Use 5 mL of M10 to wash the cells from the plate, pipetting up and down to detach remaining cells.
5. Centrifuge the resuspension (total of 8 mL) at 1000 rpm for 5 min.
6. Fill a 50 mL reservoir with 42.5 mL of M10 PSF (*see* **Note 2**).
7. Vacuum the supernatant from the centrifuged tube.
8. Resuspend the cell pellet in 5 mL of M10 PSF.
9. Add the resuspension to the 50 mL reservoir, and mix thoroughly by pipetting up and down.
10. Take 1.5 mL of this resuspension. and add to each well of the 6 well plates (this plan is designed to accommodate 24 wells total so 4 of these 6 well plates can be seeded).
11. Place a label adjacent to each well with numbering 1 to 24.
12. Use 10 mL to seed a new cell culture maintenance plate.
13. Incubate the plates for 24 hours at 37 C 5% CO_2.

3.2 Transfection

1. Prepare the transfection plan as shown in Table 1.
2. View the 6 well plates under a light microscope to confirm that the cells are attached and healthy.
3. Obtain two 5 mL Eppendorf tubes and fill one with 2.4 mL of MEM and the other with 2.5 mL of MEM.
4. Label two 12 well reservoirs with numbering 1 to 24.
5. In the 5 mL Eppendorf with 2.4 mL of MEM, add 2.4 ul of 100 ng/uL GFP plasmid, and mix this tube thoroughly.

Table 1
Transfection and cell staining plan with necessary controls

Tube	Transfection materials	Staining
1 – PE negative	GFP	7AAD
2 – 7AAD negative	OR51E2, GFP	Rho4D2, PE
3 – GFP negative	OR51E2	Rho4D2, PE, 7AAD
4 – Positive control	OR51E2, GFP	Rho4D2, PE, 7AAD
5 – Negative control	pCI, GFP	Rho4D2, PE, 7AAD
6 – First sample	Sample 1 OR, GFP (+/– RTP1S)	Rho4D2, PE, 7AAD
...	...	...
24 – Final sample	Sample 24 OR, GFP (+/– RTP1S)	Rho4D2, PE, 7AAD

It is recommended to use an OR that expresses well, like OR51E2, for tubes 2, 3, and 4 to ensure that the fluorophores and antibodies are functioning appropriately. Tubes 4 and 5 represent positive and negative controls respectively as tube 5 is transfected with the empty vector pCI which yields low PE readout. Receptor-transporting protein 1S (RTP1S) or other chaperone proteins can be cotransfected with ORs if desired

6. Distribute 100 uL of the GFP + MEM mixture to each of the 24 wells *except* for the GFP control well (tube 3 in Table 1) which receives 100 uL of pure MEM.
7. Add 12 uL of the OR containing plasmids (100 ng/uL) to wells 2 through 24, according to the transfection plan.
8. Add 100 uL of lipofectamine 2000 to the remaining Eppendorf with 2.5 mL MEM and mix.
9. Distribute 104 uL of this MEM + lipofectamine mix to the 24 wells.
10. Let the transfection mixture incubate for 15 min.
11. Add 1 mL of M10 to each well.
12. Remove the 6 well, seeded plates from the incubator.
13. Vacuum the growth media from each well, and then pipette the according transfection mix gently onto the wells' sides.
14. Repeat step 12 for the remaining plates.
15. Return the 6 well plates to the incubator for 24 hours.

3.3 Sample Preparation

1. View the 6 well plates under a light microscope to confirm that the cells are attached and healthy.
2. Fill two large Styrofoam boxes with ice.
3. In one box place the PBS + FBS + NaN_3 mixture (*see* **Note 3**) and one 50 mL conical tube containing an aliquot of this PBS incubation solution.

4. Label 24 5 mL round bottom polystyrene (PS) with numbering 1–24, and place them upright within the ice in one box.
5. Remove one 6 well plate from the incubator.
6. Vacuum the growth media from each well and pipette 1 mL of the PBS incubation mixture gently onto the sides of each well.
7. Vacuum the PBS incubation mixture from each well, and then pipette 1 mL of cell stripper directly onto the bottom of the well.
8. Mechanically detach the cells from each well by pipetting the cell stripper up and down, and transport the resuspended cells to their according round bottom tube on ice.
9. Use 1 mL of the PBS incubation mixture to wash any remaining cells from the wells and add to the PS tubes.
10. Centrifuge the tubes for 2 min at 4 C.
11. Prepare the primary antibody dilution in a 5 mL Eppendorf tube by adding 5 uL of the anti-rho 4D2 antibody to 2 mL of PBS incubation mixture (*see* **Note 4**).
12. Vacuum supernatant from PS tubes and resuspend each pellet in 80 uL of the antibody dilution, except for the PE negative control tube which receives only PBS incubation mixture, by pipetting up and down.
13. Incubate the resuspension on ice for 30 min.
14. Add 2 mL of PBS mixture to each tube.
15. Centrifuge the tubes for 2 min at 4 C.
16. Prepare the secondary antibody dilution in a 5 mL Eppendorf wrapped in foil by adding 10 uL of the phycoerythrin (PE) secondary antibody to 2 mL of PBS incubation mixture.
17. Vacuum supernatant from PS tubes and resuspend each pellet in 80 uL of the secondary antibody dilution, except for the PE negative control tube which receives only PBS incubation mixture, by pipetting up and down.
18. Cover with foil and Incubate resuspension on ice for 30 min.
19. Add 2 mL of PBS mixture to each tube.
20. Centrifuge the tubes for 2 min at 4 C.
21. Vacuum the supernatant from PS tubes and pipette 1 mL of the PBS incubation mixture into the tubes (no need for resuspension).
22. Centrifuge the tubes for 3 min at 4 C.
23. Prepare the 7AAD dilution in a 15 mL conical tube wrapped in foil by adding 26 uL of 7AAD to 13 mL of PBS incubation mixture.

24. Vacuum supernatant from PS tubes and resuspend each pellet in 500 uL of 7AAD dilution, except for the control tube which receives 500 uL PBS incubation mixture, by pipetting vigorously up and down.
25. Cover samples in foil and bring them to flow cytometry machine.

3.4 Flow Cytometry Gating Setup

The steps required to setup your experiment, adjust gatings, and output. FCS files will likely depend on the type of cytometer available and software version of FACSDiva; however, the theory behind our approach's gating remains consistent (*see* **Note 5**).

1. Access the FACSDiva™ software and create a new experiment.
2. In cytometer settings for this experiment, select the parameters tab, and delete all parameters aside from FSC (area and height) and SSC (area).
3. Add GFP, 7AAD, and PE (*see* **note 6**).
4. Make sure all fluorophores have area and log checkboxes selected.
5. Create a new specimen and open Tube 1.
6. Add a new dotplot with FSC-A on the X-axis and SSC-A on the Y-axis.
7. Draw a polygon gating that approximates the display in Fig. 2a to filter out debris and select cells.
8. Add a population hierarchy diagram and use this interface to rename the first gating to "Cells."
9. Add another dotplot with FSC-A on the X-axis and FSC-H on the Y-axis, and use the inspector window to select the cells from the first gating for this plot.
10. Add a polygon gate that is similar to Fig. 2b to filter out doublets, and select singlets and rename this gating accordingly.
11. Add another dotplot with 7AAD-A (*see* **Note 7**) on the X-axis and FSC-A on the Y-axis, and use the inspector window to select singlets for this plot.
12. Add a polygon gate that is similar to Fig. 2c to filter out dead/stressed cells, and select viable cells.
13. Add a dotplot with PE-A on the X-axis and GFP-A on the Y-axis, and use inspector window to select viable cells for this plot.
14. Create a rectangle gating for GFP+ cells that have been successfully transfected and rename this gating to GFP+.
15. In the acquisition dashboard, set the stopping gate to GFP+, and set the events to record to 10,000.

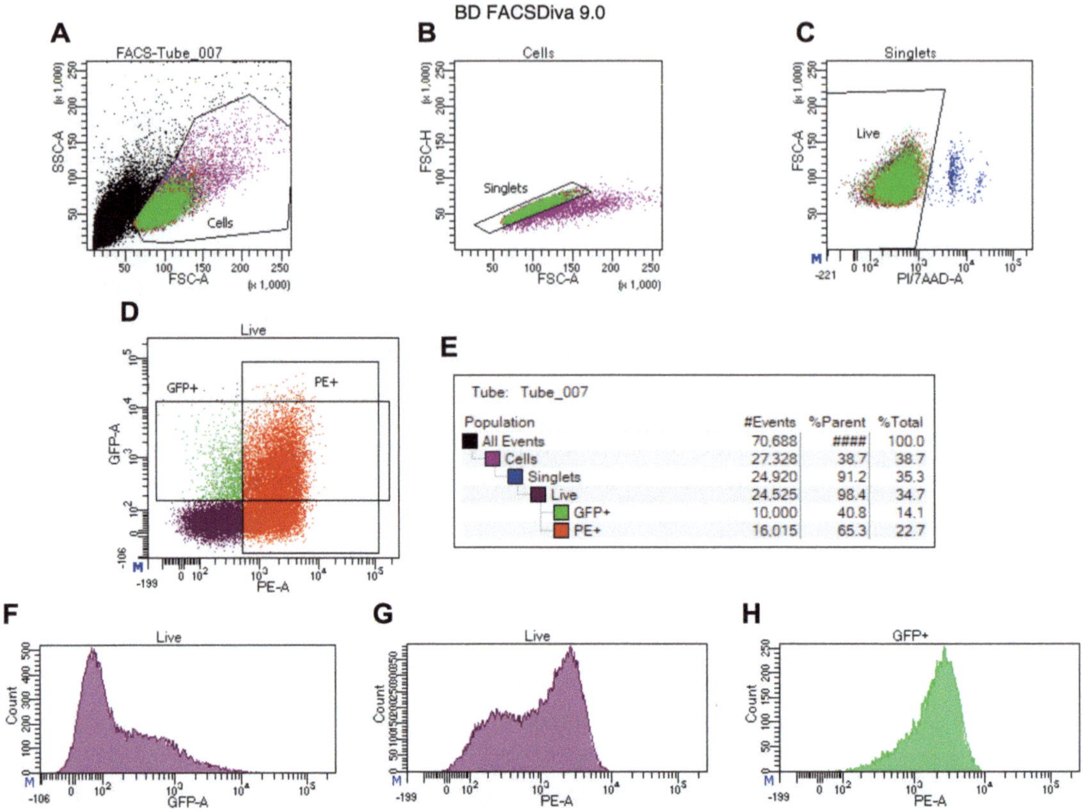

Fig. 2 FACSDiva worksheet gating selections for OR1A1 + RTP1S. (**a**) The first gating uses side-scatter area (Y-axis) and forward-scatter area (X-axis) to filter out debris, shown in black. (**b**) Secondary gating selects singlets and filters out doublets and other cellular aggregates, shown in purple, using forward scatter height (Y-axis) and forward scatter area (X-axis). (**c**) 7AAD viability nuclear staining is used to filter out dead cells, shown in blue. High 7AAD values on the log scale X-axis indicate cell membrane permeabilization which serves as a marker for cell death. (**d**) Gating to select cells that are GFP positive or PE positive. (**e**) Display of the gating hierarchy and the percentages of cells passing through each gate. (**f** and **g**) Outputs of the GFP+ and PE+ gating are useful visualizations if there are errors in transfection or antibody binding. The GFP+ gating provides the population of 10,000 cells used for PE quantification (h) which is a measurement of cell surface expression

16. At this point, the gating schema should select for and measure PE emission of single cells with detectable GFP fluorescence and low 7AAD fluorescence.
17. Additional parameters and gatings can be added like the PE+ to facilitate retrospective gating which is displayed in Fig. 2g; however, this is up to each user's discretion.

3.5 Sample Reading

1. Vortex and load your first tube which should be PE negative (if following the transfection plan provided in Table 1), and click "record data."

2. After a sufficient number cells are acquired, click "stop acquiring" and remove the tube.
3. Adjust the first and second gatings to filter out debris and doublets.
4. Vortex and record the next tube which should be 7AAD negative.
5. Adjust the gating of the viable cells (Fig. 2c) such that the polygon is including the entire population of cells from this tube.
6. After 10,000 cells are acquired, vortex and load the next tube which is GFP negative.
7. Move the GFP+ gating upward so that fewer than 0.5% of cells from this tube are captured.
8. After a sufficient number of cells are recorded, stop acquiring.
9. Vortex and load tube 4 which should contain a positive control (a well expressed OR) and collect 10,000 GFP positive cells.
10. Repeat step 9 for the remaining tubes.
11. After collection, click the experiment, select "export .FCS files," and export the experimental data to the desired folder.

3.6 Analysis

Alternatives to the software we use, FlowJo, will likely change how analysis is performed but the theory applied in our method is translatable to other pipelines. Additionally, because most of the gating is performed during collection, the analysis is relatively simple although one can opt to export all processed events from the cytometer and perform gating post collection.

1. Rename the .FCS files according to your transfection plan and open them in FlowJo.
2. Access the "layout editor" tab, and drag cell populations of interest into this new sheet.
3. Change the X and Y axes to display values of interest like PE-A and count as shown in Fig. 3.
4. To quantify cell surface expression, right-click your sample and select "Add Statistic" and select geometric mean of PE.
5. Right-click the resulting value and apply it to all sample tubes.

4 Notes

1. The rho-tag sequence, derived from the N-terminal sequence of bovine rhodopsin, is " MNGTEGPNFYVPFSNKTGVV." Alternative epitopes and antibodies like the flag-tag and anti-flag M2 can be substituted if preferred.

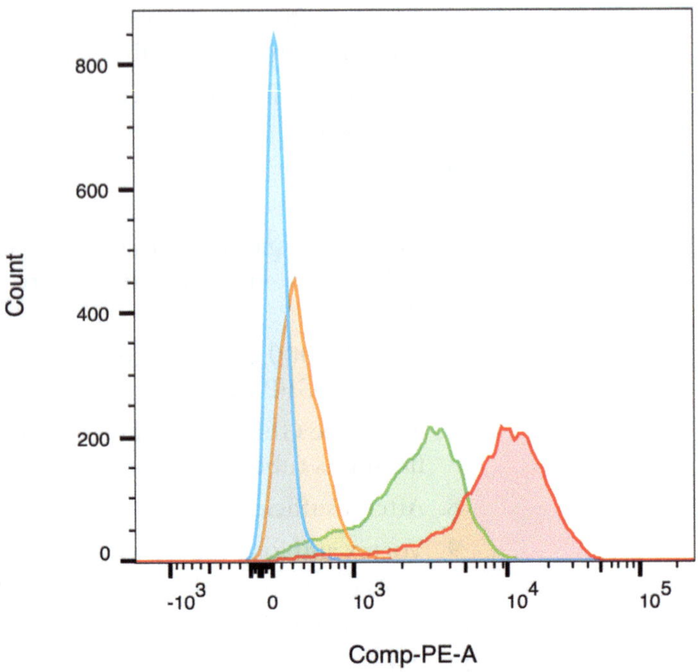

	Sample Name	Geometric Mean : Comp-PE-A
(red)	OR51E2_Tube_004.fcs	8102
(blue)	pCI_Tube_005.fcs	186
(orange)	OR1A1_Tube_006.fcs	414
(green)	OR1A1_+RTP1S_Tube_007.fcs	2281

Fig. 3 Phycoerythrin histograms quantifying cell surface expression. The X-axis represents PE emission signal intensity while the X-axis indicates the number of cells. The empty pCI vector (blue) is used as a negative control, whereas the highly expressed OR51E2 (red) is used as a positive control. OR1A1 shows improvement when cotransfected with RTP1S as demonstrated by a rightward shift in its histogram (orange to green). The geometric mean of the PE value can be used as a numeric summary of these expression histograms

2. This resuspension volume can be adjusted to accommodate different numbers of samples. Our protocol allows for the seeding of four 6-well plates (24 wells total) with 1.5 mL of the resuspension in each well and the remaining 10 mL of resuspension for continuing the cell line.
3. It is easiest to add 10 mL FBS and 5 mL 1.5 M sodium azide directly to a container with 500 mL PBS and place this container on ice, taking aliquots into the 50 mL conical (also on ice) to use for pipetting.
4. This dilution varies depending on the antibody used, for anti-rho 4D2, we have found that 1/400 dilution is most efficient, whereas for anti-flag M2, 1/600 is optimal.

5. We recommend setting up the BD FACSDiva experimental parameters on your cytometer computer prior to running the first experiment, so there is minimal waiting time between 7AAD staining and detection.
6. Voltages and compensation values should be preset; otherwise you will have to perform a calibration experiment which is beyond the scope of this protocol.
7. Biexponential plots should be enabled for the dotplots of the different fluorophores to allow visualization of negative values. This can be accessed in the plot tab of the inspector panel.
8. PE values can fluctuate between experiments; thus it is best practice to normalize by positive or negative controls instead of comparing raw geometric mean PEs. Alternatively one could use nonparametric comparisons like ranking to compare between experiments [6].

References

1. Malnic B, Godfrey PA, Buck LB (2004) The Human olfactory receptor gene family. Proceedings of the National Academy of Sciences USA 101:2584–2589
2. Malnic B, Hirono J, Sato T, Buck LB (1996) Combinatorial receptor codes for odors. Cell 96: 713–723
3. Glusman G, Yanai I, Rubin I, Lancet D (2001) The complete human olfactory subgenome. Genome Res 11:685–702
4. Ikegami K, de March CA, Nagai MH, Ghosh S, Do M, Sharma R, Bruguera ES, Lu YE, Fukutani Y, Nagarajan V, Yohda M, Matsunami H (2020) Structural instability and divergence from conserved residues underlie intracellular retention of mammalian odorant receptors. Proceedings of the National Academy of Sciences USA 117:2957–2967
5. Saito H, Kubota M, Roberts RW, Chi Q, Matsunami H (2004) RTP family members induce functional expression of mammalian odorant receptors. Cell 119:679–691
6. Billesbolle CB, de March CA, van der Velden WJC, Ning M, Tewari J, del Torrent CL, Li L, Faust B, Vaidehi N, Matsunami H, Manglik A (2023) Structural basis of odorant recognition by a human odorant receptor. Nature 615:742–749

Chapter 9

Dissociation of Mouse Olfactory Mucosae for Fluorescence-Activated Cell Sorting of Olfactory Sensory Neurons

Qiang Wang, Tomoko Sengoku, William B. Titlow, Jennifer L. Strange, and Timothy S. McClintock

Abstract

An increasing diversity of techniques investigating the biology of specific cell types and individual cells have elevated the importance of dissociation of viable cells from living tissues. Here we describe a method for the dissociation of single cells from samples of adult mouse olfactory mucosae, with an emphasis on maximizing yield of viable single cells from fluorescence-activated cell sorting. Yields are typically in the range of 80,000–150,000 viable cells per adult mouse.

Key words FACS, Olfaction, Single-cell RNA-seq, GFP, Smell, RNA-seq, ChIP-seq

1 Introduction

The need to isolate live cells from the vertebrate olfactory epithelium has grown along with technological advances that require single cells or purified samples of specific cell types and cell subtypes. The advent of patch clamp electrophysiology spurred the development of methods to disperse olfactory mucosae into single cells [1]. The ability to make genetically modified mice carrying reporter genes, especially green fluorescent protein (GFP) [2, 3], allowed the isolation of reliably identified cell types from the olfactory epithelium and stimulated efforts to isolate olfactory epithelium cells from live mice [4, 5]. Molecular characterizations of olfactory epithelium cell types followed, especially transcriptome measurement and chromatin-immunoprecipitation sequencing (ChIP-seq) experiments focused on individual cell types [4–9]. Next came single-cell RNA-seq experiments that identify the most common mRNAs in individual cells, thereby providing measures of changes in phenotype (e.g., development) and relative proportions

Bradley J. Goldstein and Hiroaki Matsunami (eds.), *The Olfactory System*, Methods in Molecular Biology, vol. 2710, https://doi.org/10.1007/978-1-0716-3425-7_9,

of cell types and subtypes [10–13]. The past several years have seen continued expansion of projects using dissociation of olfactory mucosa as one of their fundamental methods [8, 9, 14–16].

The procedure we describe here has a long history. It began as a method to isolate vomeronasal sensory neurons for electrophysiological recording of responses to pheromones, experiments that require a gentle approach yielding neurons with intact (or nearly intact) dendrites and cilia [17]. We iteratively modified it for olfactory sensory neurons (OSNs), to increase the yield of viable cells, to minimize opportunity for changes in gene expression, and to be better suited for fluorescence-activated cell sorting (FACS) [4–6, 18, 19]. Modifications were incorporated into the method when they improved cell survival, measured via flow cytometry or FACS as the number of viable cells per mouse, the number of GFP^+ OSNs per mouse, or the amount of total RNA in samples of GFP^+ OSNs. Though emphasis throughout has been to isolate OSNs, all olfactory epithelium cell types survive in sufficient numbers to have their specific markers detected in downstream analyses.

2 Materials

2.1 Solutions

1. Hank's Balanced Salt Solution (HBSS). Store working stock at 4 °C. Additional bottles can be stored at room temperature.
2. Low Calcium Saline. Make working stock solutions listed in Table 1. Store the glucose stock solution at 4 °C, the others at room temperature. Mix the stock solution volumes indicated in

Table 1
Stock solutions, formula, and composition of Low Calcium Saline

Component	Stock solution (M)	Volume of stock (mL)	Final concentration (mM)
NaCl	1	22	110
$NaHCO_3$	1	5	25
KCl	1	1	5
N,N-bis(2-hydroxyethyl)-2-aminoethanesulfonic acid (BES)	1	1	5
$MgSO_4$	1	0.2	1
$CaCl_2$	1	0.96	4.8
EGTA	0.5	2	5
NaOH	1	2	10
D-Glucose	1	2	10

Table 1 with ultrapure water to reach 200 mL. Pass through a 0.22 μm filter. The pH of this solution is ~9. Store at 4 °C.

3. Oxygenated Low Calcium Saline. No more than 24 h prior to use, bubble oxygen through a bottle of Low Calcium Saline until the pH reaches ~6.5 as indicated by pH paper. This can take 1–2 h.
4. 1.5 M cysteine.

2.2 Enzymes

1. Papain from papaya latex, 10 U/mg. Store at 4–20 °C.
2. Trypsin from porcine pancreas, 20,000 U/mg. Store at −20 °C.
3. DNase I (RNase free), 2 U/μL. Store at −20 °C.

2.3 Sorting

1. 8 peak alignment rainbow beads.
2. Sheath fluid of choice.

3 Methods

This procedure is designed to produce four pooled samples of dissociated cells, each pool consisting of the olfactory mucosae from three mice. The sequential production of four pooled samples, FACS of these samples, and the RNA isolation that typically follows requires an entire workday.

3.1 Preparations

1. Cool benchtop centrifuge to 4 °C.
2. Weigh out 4.2 mg papain and dissolve in 3 mL of oxygenated Low Calcium Saline. Add 1.5 μL of DNase I. Lastly, add 10 μL of 1.5 M cysteine that has been heated at 95 °C for >10 min. Incubate at 37 °C for ~10 min to ensure papain is completely dissolved in solution. Store on ice.
3. Weigh out 6.0 mg trypsin and dissolve in 3 mL of (non-oxygenated) Low Calcium Saline. Add 1.5 μL of DNase I. Store on ice.
4. Make two 45 mL aliquots of HBSS, add 45 μL of DNAse I to each aliquot and place on ice.

3.2 Dissociation of Olfactory Mucosae

1. Dissect olfactory mucosae from a freshly euthanized mouse, placing the tissue into a 2 mL collection tube containing 700 μL of ice-cold oxygenated Low Calcium Saline. Do this separately for each mouse (*see* **Note 1**).
2. Homogenize the tissue using a disposable plastic tip on a rotor-stator type homogenizer at the device's lowest setting. Homogenize for 50–60 s, slowly rotating the tube. Do not

allow the tip to withdraw from the solution until the tip has come to full stop (*see* **Note 2**).

3. Using a 1 mL pipette tip that has been cut back by ~1 cm, transfer the homogenized tissue into a precooled 1.5 mL tube.
4. Add 150 μL of the papain solution, close the tube, and mix by inverting (*see* **Note 3**).
5. Incubate at 37 °C for 15 min.
6. Add 450 μL of the trypsin solution, mix by inverting (*see* **Note 4**).
7. Incubate at 37 °C for 5 min.
8. Transfer into a 13 × 100 mm glass culture tube containing 3 mL of cold HBSS containing DNase I (*see* **Note 5**).
9. Homogenize the tissue using a disposable plastic tip on a rotor-stator type homogenizer at the device's lowest setting. Homogenize for 20 s, slowly rotating the tube. Do not allow the tip to withdraw from the solution until the tip has come to full stop (*see* **Note 6**).
10. Centrifuge at 200× *g* for 10 min at 4 °C.
11. Carefully decant the supernatant (*see* **Note 7**).
12. Add 3 mL of cold HBSS containing DNase I.
13. Homogenize the tissue using a disposable plastic tip on a rotor-stator type homogenizer at the device's lowest setting. Homogenize for 20 s, slowly rotating the tube. Do not allow the tip to withdraw from the solution until the tip has come to full stop.
14. Centrifuge at 200× *g* for 10 min at 4 °C.
15. Carefully decant the supernatant.
16. Add 800 μL of cold HBSS containing DNase I. Gently triturate twice with a 1 mL tip and then vortex for 2 sec.
17. Filter the cells by applying the cell suspension to a 5 mL polystyrene round-bottom tube with cell-strainer cap (35 μm mesh) using a 1 mL pipet (*see* **Note 8**).
18. Add 3 μL of DNase I and incubate at 37 °C for 2 min.
19. Filter the cells again by applying them to a 5 mL polystyrene round-bottom tube with cell-strainer cap (35 μm mesh) using a 1 mL pipet (*see* **Note 9**).
20. Pooling. Samples can be pooled after filtering separately, or by filtering samples sequentially through the same strainer cap.
21. Place tubes on ice. For samples destined for FACS, add 6 μL of propidium iodide (PI) (1 mg/mL), and mix.

3.3 Optimization, Calibration, and Standardization of the Cell Sorter

1. Set up a flow cytometer equipped with lasers for GFP and propidium iodide (PI). Use a 100 micron nozzle tip at 15 psi (*see* **Note 10**).
2. Set the circulating chiller at 4 °C to keep the samples and collection tubes at a constant temperature.
3. Perform manual alignment. Set sort drop delay and calculate laser time delays using calibration beads. Then optimize the manual alignment of the sorter with eight peak alignment rainbow beads (*see* **Note 11**).
4. Optimize fluorescence channels using the eight peak alignment beads. A 525/50 nm emission filter is used for GFP fluorescence and excited off the 488 nm laser. For cell viability detection via PI use 561 nm laser excitation with a 585/40 nm emission filter. PI labeling of DNA identifies dead cells during FACS.
5. Set a forward-scatter (size) versus side-scatter (granularity) plot window to distinguish viable cells from debris and dead cells, which have smaller size and more granularity than live cells (*see* **Note 12**).
6. Set a forward-scatter height versus forward-scatter area plot window for doublet discrimination.
7. Set a two-color dot plot to reflect GFP (525/50 blue area) versus PI (585/40 green area) fluorescence.
8. Acquire ~10,000 events at 250 events/sec of the eight peak alignment beads (Fig. 1a). Adjust photomultiplier tube (PMT) voltage as needed to standardize the fluorescence of the eight peak beads (Fig. 1b).
9. Acquire a few thousand events from a dispersed cell sample. Use forward-scatter versus side-scatter window to identify a region of viable cells (Fig. 2a, b), and gate them.
10. Gate single cells based on the forward-scatter height versus forward-scatter area window (Fig. 2c, d).
11. To establish the upper end of cell autofluorescence use samples lacking GFP, such as from wild-type mice (e.g., Fig. 2e), to determine where autofluorescence is located. Use the upper limit of autofluorescence to set GFP-positive and GFP-negative region gates. Once this has been done for several samples on several different days to confirm that this boundary is stable, it is no longer necessary to test wild-type samples every time sorting is done. Instead, the position of this boundary can be located in the eight peak alignment bead distribution (Fig. 1b). Use this now standardized limit of sample autofluorescence to set two gating regions, one for GFP negative cells and one for GFP positive cells. Set regions to exclude all cells positive for PI (Fig. 2e, f) (*see* **Note 13**).

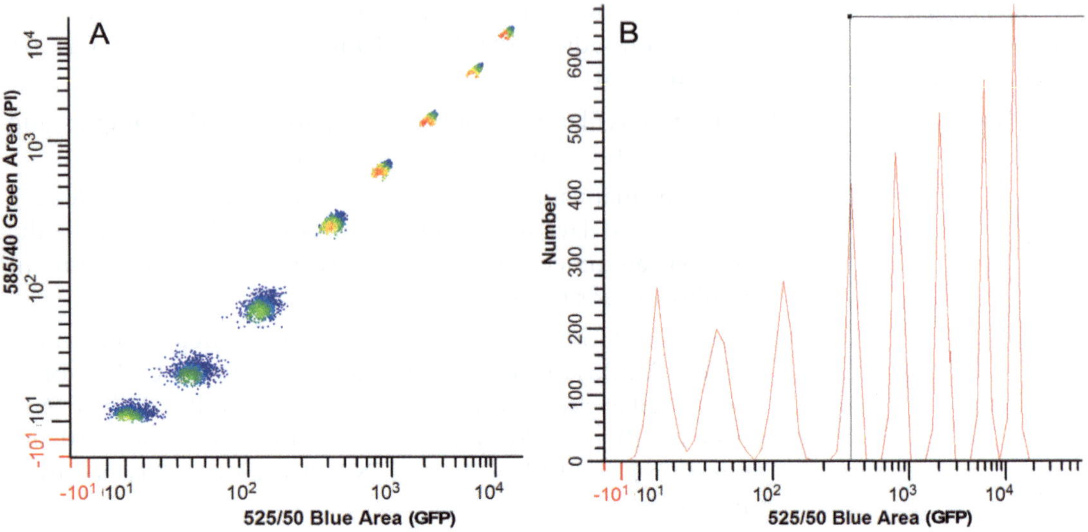

Fig. 1 Setting the gate between GFP fluorescent and nonfluorescent cells. We discovered empirically that the fourth peak in the eight peak bead FACS standard sits at the upper end of cell autofluorescence. Using this peak to set the gate avoids variation in gate position due to differences in the number of autofluorescent cells between samples, a problem discovered when using dissociated olfactory mucosae from wild-type mice to set the gate. (**a**) The distribution of eight peak alignment rainbow beads. (**b**) The distribution of the peaks of the eight peak alignment beads with the boundary between the GFP negative and positive regions superimposed

12. Set sort mode to purify.
13. Sort samples at a rate of 1500 cells/s.
14. For samples destined for isolation of total RNA, sort directly into the cell lysis buffer of your preferred RNA isolation method. Otherwise, sort into fetal bovine serum or the culture medium of choice (*see* **Note 14**).

4 Notes

1. Better yields are obtained if the olfactory mucosa from each mouse is carried through the procedure separately before pooling (three mice per pool) at the second filtering step, as we describe in this protocol.
2. We have only ever used an Omni GLH-115 General Laboratory Homogenizer with a disposable Hard Tissue Omni Tip (Omni International, 30750H, 7 × 110 mm) at a speed setting of 1 for this step. Other rotor-stator homogenizers that have disposable plastic tips should suffice, but users will need to do pilot tests to optimize speed setting and duration. Homogenization times in the range of 20–60 sec give yields equivalent to 120 sec and twice that of 6 sec. The disposable

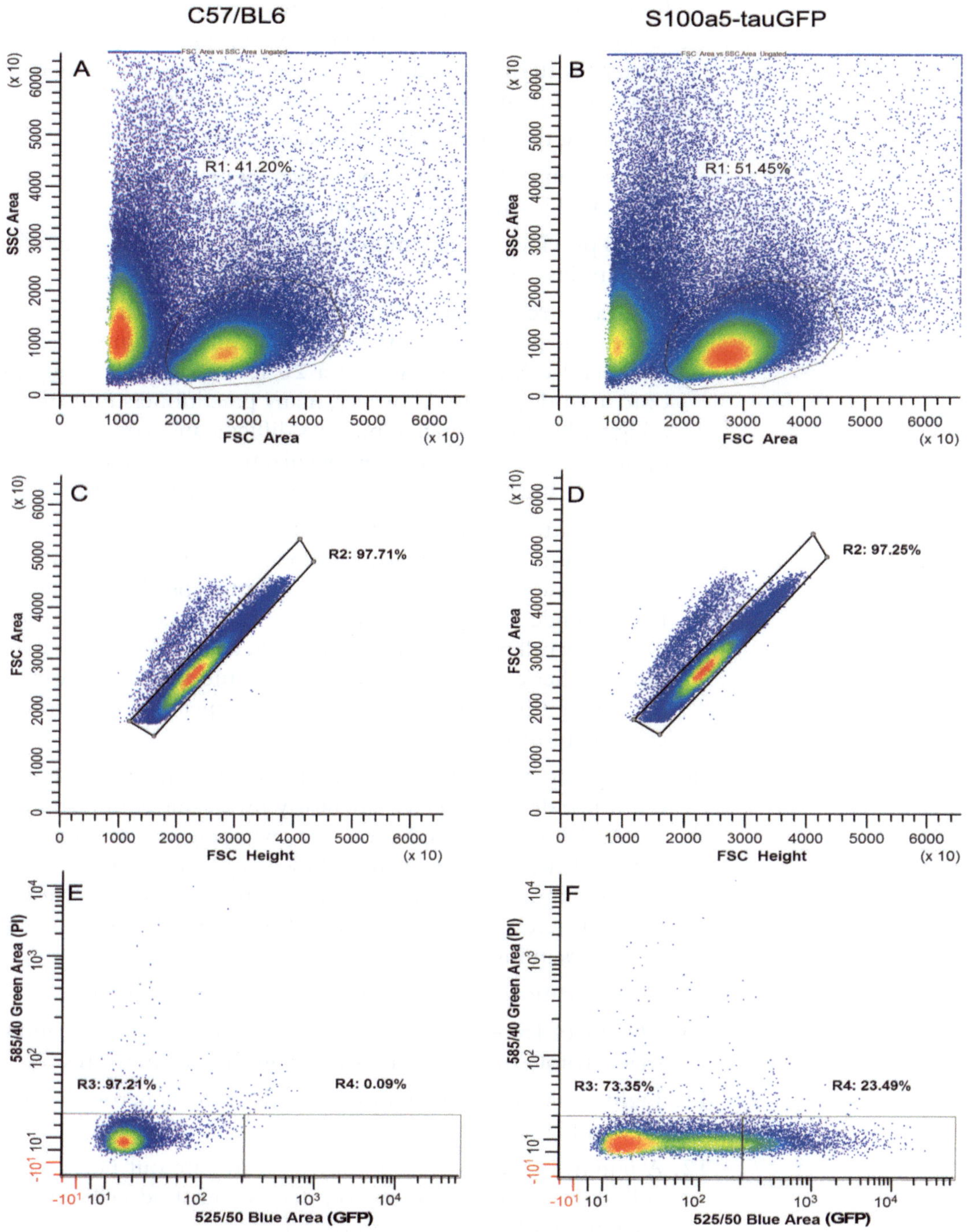

Fig. 2 FACS of dissociated olfactory mucosae from a wild-type C57/BL6 sample and a *S100a5-tauGFP*$^{(+/-)}$ sample. (**a** and **b**) Forward-scatter versus side-scatter plot identifies viable cells (R1 gates). (**c** and **d**) Forward-scatter area versus height applied to the R1 gate to discriminate single cells from cell clusters. (**e** and **f**) Fluorescence plot of cells in the R2 gate to discriminate GFP$^+$ OSNs (R4 gate) from GFP$^-$ cells (R3 gate)

homogenization tips should be swapped out between each sample, though samples destined to be pooled can be homogenized with the same tip. These disposable tips can be cleaned and reused many times without affecting outcomes.

3. Increasing the concentration of papain does not improve yield.
4. The trypsin step may be superfluous. Some practitioners have eliminated it without significant effects on yield.
5. HBSS provides a small improvement over the saline originally used in this procedure.
6. Equivalent results can be obtained by gently triturating instead of homogenizing at steps 9 and 13 of Subheading 3.2 to resuspend cell pellets. We use a 20 μL pipette tip snugly fit onto a 1 mL pipette. However, many practitioners find triturating without introducing bubbles difficult and slower, instead opting for the low-speed homogenization. Tests of trituration using a syringe and 26 gauge needle gave inferior yields.
7. Do not attempt to decant repeatedly or to remove all the supernatant. The ~100 μL of supernatant remaining after a typical decant will not affect subsequent steps. The cell pellet from a single mouse is difficult to see. If there is concern about loss of the cell pellet in steps 11 and 15, decant the supernatant into another culture tube and store this tube on ice. However, once decanting without "wash back" of supernatant is learned, cell pellet loss is avoided.
8. Cell aggregations, slow filtering, sticky solutions, and clogging of the nozzle during FACS are nearly always due to undegraded DNA. Adding more DNase I and switching to a fresh vial of DNase I nearly always solves these problems. In the case of nozzle clogging the sample can be rescued by adding DNase I, doing a quick vortex, and incubating at 37 °C for 2–5 min before resuming the sort.
9. Centrifugation at 200× *g* can be done to speed filtering.
10. The use of 15 psi significantly improves yield over 30 psi, more than twofold in some tests comparing the two pressures.
11. Eight peak alignment rainbow beads from Spherotech were used in Fig. 1.
12. A minimal threshold is typically used to gate out noise while still allowing sort decisions on debris and dead cells so that accurate purity values are produced.
13. Two different strains of mice whose OSNs express GFP show the same autofluorescence pattern and therefore require the same gating edge position in the eight peak alignment bead distribution (the center of the fourth peak), indicating that this

location is broadly applicable. Nevertheless, verifying this with each new strain is good practice.

14. Polypropylene tubes are best for collection of sorted cells. Tube size depends on the number of cells being collected per tube. For RNA isolation the volume collected is typically determined by the amount of dilution of cell lysis buffer allowed by the RNA isolation procedure. For 100 μm nozzle tips, each droplet is approximately 3 nL.

References

1. Firestein S, Werblin F (1989) Odor-induced membrane currents in vertebrate-olfactory receptor neurons. Science 244:79–82. https://doi.org/10.1126/science.2704991
2. Mombaerts P, Wang F, Dulac C, Chao SK, Nemes A, Mendelsohn M, Edmondson J, Axel R (1996) Visualizing an olfactory sensory map. Cell 87:675–686
3. Potter SM, Zheng C, Koos DS, Feinstein P, Fraser SE, Mombaerts P (2001) Structure and emergence of specific olfactory glomeruli in the mouse. J Neurosci 21:9713–9723
4. Sammeta N, Yu TT, Bose SC, McClintock TS (2007) Mouse olfactory sensory neurons express 10,000 genes. J Comp Neurol 502: 1138–1156
5. Yu TT, McIntyre JC, Bose SC, Hardin D, Owen MC, McClintock TS (2005) Differentially expressed transcripts from phenotypically identified olfactory sensory neurons. J Comp Neurol 483:251–262
6. Nickell MD, Breheny P, Stromberg AJ, McClintock TS (2012) Genomics of mature and immature olfactory sensory neurons. J Comp Neurol 520:2608–2609. https://doi.org/10.1002/cne.23052
7. Ibarra-Soria X, Levitin MO, Saraiva LR, Logan DW (2014) The olfactory transcriptomes of mice. PLoS Genet 10:e1004593. https://doi.org/10.1371/journal.pgen.1004593
8. Colquitt BM, Markenscoff-Papadimitriou E, Duffie R, Lomvardas S (2014) Dnmt3a regulates global gene expression in olfactory sensory neurons and enables odorant-induced transcription. Neuron 83:823–838. https://doi.org/10.1016/j.neuron.2014.07.013
9. Magklara A, Yen A, Colquitt BM, Clowney EJ, Allen W, Markenscoff-Papadimitriou E, Evans ZA, Kheradpour P, Mountoufaris G, Carey C, Barnea G, Kellis M, Lomvardas S (2011) An epigenetic signature for monoallelic olfactory receptor expression. Cell 145:555–570. doi: S0092–8674(11)00374–6 [pii] https://doi.org/10.1016/j.cell.2011.03.040
10. Fletcher RB, Das D, Gadye L, Street KN, Baudhuin A, Wagner A, Cole MB, Flores Q, Choi YG, Yosef N, Purdom E, Dudoit S, Risso D, Ngai J (2017) Deconstructing olfactory stem cell trajectories at single-cell resolution. Cell Stem Cell 20:817-830 e8. https://doi.org/10.1016/j.stem.2017.04.003
11. Hanchate NK, Kondoh K, Lu Z, Kuang D, Ye X, Qiu X, Pachter L, Trapnell C, Buck LB (2015) Single-cell transcriptomics reveals receptor transformations during olfactory neurogenesis. Science 350:1251–1255. https://doi.org/10.1126/science.aad2456
12. Saraiva LR, Ibarra-Soria X, Khan M, Omura M, Scialdone A, Mombaerts P, Marioni JC, Logan DW (2015) Hierarchical deconstruction of mouse olfactory sensory neurons: from whole mucosa to single-cell RNA-seq. Sci Rep 5: 18178. https://doi.org/10.1038/srep18178
13. Tan L, Li Q, Xie XS (2015) Olfactory sensory neurons transiently express multiple olfactory receptors during development. Mol Syst Biol 11:844. https://doi.org/10.15252/msb.20156639
14. Horgue LF, Assens A, Fodoulian L, Marconi L, Tuberosa J, Haider A, Boillat M, Carleton A, Rodriguez I (2022) Transcriptional adaptation of olfactory sensory neurons to GPCR identity and activity. Nat Commun 13:2929. https://doi.org/10.1038/s41467-022-30511-4
15. Shayya HJ, Kahiapo JK, Duffie R, Lehmann KS, Bashkirova L, Monahan K, Dalton RP, Gao J, Jiao S, Schieren I, Belluscio L, Lomvardas S (2022) ER stress transforms random olfactory receptor choice into axon targeting precision. Cell. https://doi.org/10.1016/j.cell.2022.08.025
16. Tsukahara T, Brann DH, Pashkovski SL, Guitchounts G, Bozza T, Datta SR (2021) A transcriptional rheostat couples past activity to future sensory responses. Cell 184:6326-6343 e32. https://doi.org/10.1016/j.cell.2021.11.022

17. Lucas P, Ukhanov K, Leinders-Zufall T, Zufall F (2003) A diacylglycerol-gated cation channel in vomeronasal neuron dendrites is impaired in TRPC2 mutant mice: mechanism of pheromone transduction. Neuron 40:551–561
18. de March CA, Titlow WB, Sengoku T, Breheny P, Matsunami H, McClintock TS (2020) Modulation of the combinatorial code of odorant receptor response patterns in odorant mixtures. Mol Cell Neurosci 104:103469. https://doi.org/10.1016/j.mcn.2020.103469
19. McClintock TS, Adipietro K, Titlow WB, Breheny P, Walz A, Mombaerts P, Matsunami H (2014) In vivo identification of eugenol-responsive and muscone-responsive mouse odorant receptors. J Neurosci 34:15669–15678. https://doi.org/10.1523/JNEUROSCI.3625-14.2014

Chapter 10

Preparation of Human Olfactory Epithelial Biopsies for Downstream Analysis

Rhea Choi, Tiffany Ko, John B. Finlay, Ralph Abi Hachem, David Jang, and Bradley J. Goldstein

Abstract

The olfactory mucosa, lining a portion of the nasal cavity, houses the primary olfactory sensory neurons responsible for odor transduction, along with supporting cell populations. Tremendous advances have come from studying the peripheral olfactory system in animal models, especially the mouse. However, acquired human olfactory disorders lack effective therapies, and many of these conditions involve pathology in the olfactory mucosa. Thus, the ability to obtain human olfactory biopsy samples from subjects with olfactory dysfunction, or controls, may be of value. Here, we describe established techniques for collecting olfactory tissue from human subjects and preparing samples for downstream assays such as immunohistochemistry, flow cytometry, single-cell RNA-sequencing, or chromatin studies.

Key words Human olfactory epithelium, Olfactory cleft, Endoscopic endonasal approach, Nasal cytology

1 Introduction

Animal models are the most widely used systems to study olfactory neurobiology. For instance, mouse genetic systems enabling lineage tracing and/or gene deletion can be coupled with experimental injuries such as olfactory bulb ablation or chemical lesion, to enable study of specific cell populations or gene function in normal or regenerating olfactory epithelium [1]. While there are many similarities between mouse and human olfactory epithelium, the translation of discoveries into new treatments for human olfactory disorders may benefit from an ability to examine human olfactory cells, from both normal and diseased subjects. The location of the olfactory epithelium at the lining of the nasal airspace (Fig. 1) provides a unique opportunity to biopsy, from live patients, this peripheral neurosensory structure [2–4].

Bradley J. Goldstein and Hiroaki Matsunami (eds.), *The Olfactory System*, Methods in Molecular Biology, vol. 2710, https://doi.org/10.1007/978-1-0716-3425-7_10,

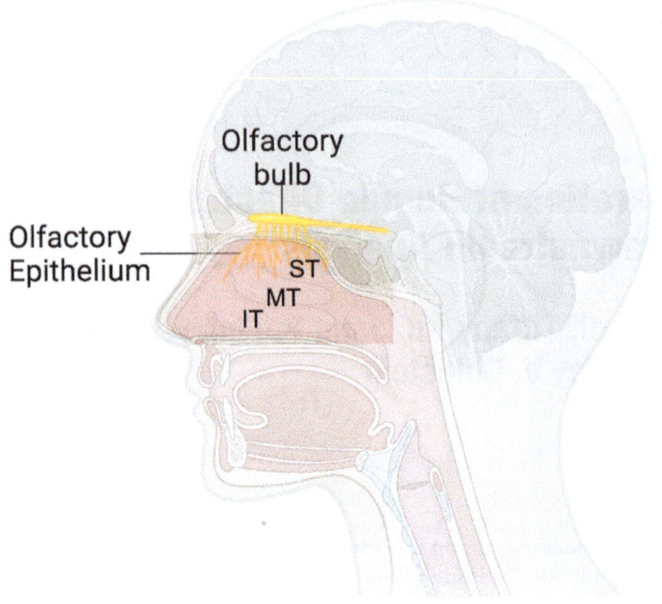

Fig. 1 Olfactory cleft anatomy. Schematic representation of the lateral nasal wall. The olfactory epithelium is limited to the yellow labeled area in the superior nasal cavity, along portions of the superior turbinate (ST) and middle turbinate (MT), and the corresponding superior nasal septum. The remainder of the nasal cavity, including the inferior turbinate (IT), is lined by respiratory epithelium lacking olfactory neurons. The neurons of the olfactory epithelium project axons as cranial nerve I through the cribriform plate to synapse at the olfactory bulbs of the brain

This chapter describes techniques to obtain and process human olfactory tissue for downstream assays. The olfactory mucosa consists of a surface neuroepithelium housing sustentacular cells, microvillar cells, olfactory sensory neurons, and basal cells and an underlying lamina propria consisting of Bowman's glands, olfactory axon fascicles with surrounding olfactory ensheathing glia, blood vessels, and fibroblasts [5, 6]. Immune cells are also present in both the lamina propria and surface epithelium. In humans, the olfactory mucosa is located within a very limited region of the nasal cavity called the olfactory cleft. The olfactory cleft is situated along the superior medial vertical lamella of the superior turbinate, a similar small portion of the middle turbinate, and the corresponding nasal septum [7]. The remainder of the nasal cavity is lined with a respiratory surface epithelium, although the distribution of respiratory versus olfactory epithelium can vary based on age and other factors. Sinonasal infection, inflammation, or other pathology could affect the epithelial distribution (respiratory vs. olfactory), quality, and biology of the tissue samples. Endoscopic nasal surgeries have provided an opportunity to obtain olfactory cleft biopsies for research [8–10]. For instance, patients undergoing endoscopic endonasal trans-sphenoid approaches for resection of anterior skull base or pituitary tumors often have no pathology involving the nasal epithelium and require resection of at least limited portions of the olfactory cleft to provide surgical access to the tumor. Also, office based endoscopic biopsy approaches can be performed in appropriate subjects [11–13]. In all cases, biopsies must be obtained in accordance with specific approved Institutional Review Board (IRB) protocols.

2 Materials

2.1 Instruments/Supplies for Collecting Surgical Olfactory Mucosa Biopsy

1. 4 mm 0 degree or 30 degree rigid nasal endoscope with camera attachment and video monitor (Karl Storz or equivalent).
2. #12 blade and blade handle.
3. Oxymetazoline hydrochloride 0.05% with 1% lidocaine.
4. Cotton pledgets.
5. Cottle or freer elevator.
6. Small straight through-cutting ethmoid forceps.
7. Collection solution: Hanks' balanced salt solution (HBSS) or Hibernate E.
8. Collection tube, such as 15 ml polystyrene Falcon tube.

2.2 Instruments/Supplies for Collecting Cytology Biopsy

1. 4 mm 0 degree or 30 degree rigid nasal endoscope with camera attachment and video monitor (Karl Storz or equivalent).
2. Oxymetazoline hydrochloride 0.05% with 1% lidocaine.
3. Nasal cytology brush (we use catalog no. 4290, Hobbs Medical Inc., Stafford Springs, CT).
4. HBSS or Hibernate E.
5. Collection tube, such as 15 ml polystyrene Falcon tube.

2.3 Tissue Dissociation

1. Enzyme cocktail 1: 1 U/ml dispase, 1 mg/ml collagenase A, and 0.1 mg/ml deoxyribonuclease I (DNase) in Ca/Mg-free HBSS.
2. Enzyme cocktail 2: 5 mg/ml papain diluted into 1X Accutase solution (Note: EDTA activates papain, and we use Accutase solution from StemCell Tech which contains 0.5 mM EDTA).
3. Ca/Mg-free HBSS.
4. Additional 1 mg/ml DNase 1 stock (store as 100 μl aliquots at −20°).
5. Resuspension solution: HBSS with 1 mg/ml nonacetylated bovine serum albumin (Thermo Fisher Scientific), anti-clumping reagent (0.5–1 μl/ml; Gibco).

6. Fetal bovine serum (FBS).
7. ACK lysing solution.
8. Swinging bucket refrigerated centrifuge.
9. Tissue rocker.
10. 250 μm, 70 μm, and 40 μm mesh filters.
11. Cell counter; we recommend the Cellometer K2 fluorescent counter from Nexcelom for rapid and accurate live/dead cell identification and quantification. Alternatively, Trypan Blue dye exclusion and a Neubauer hemacytometer may be used.

2.4 Processing for Frozen Section Immunohistochemistry

1. 4% paraformaldehyde in PBS or 3.7% formalin (diluted 1:10 from 37% formalin in PBS).
2. PBS.
3. Cryomold.
4. Optimal cutting temperature embedding medium (O.C.T.).
5. Cryoprotection/decalcification solution: 30% sucrose, 250 mM EDTA, PBS.
6. Liquid nitrogen.
7. Cryostat.
8. Superfrost Plus microscope slides.

2.5 Instruments or Kits for Potential Downstream Assays

1. Single-cell RNA-sequencing: we have used the 3′ gene expression kits and Chromium Controller for cell capture, RNA isolation, and barcoding, from 10X Genomics per manufacturer's instructions.
2. RNA isolation and RT-qPCR: we have used the spin column RNAmicro kit from Zymo or RNEasy kits from Qiagen per manufacturer's instruction, followed by the SuperScipt IV reverse transcription kit from Invitrogen per instructions to generate cDNA for qPCR template.
3. Spectrophotometer for DNA or RNA quantification (e.g., NanoDrop, Thermo Fisher).

3 Methods

All human samples should be collected and stored according to an approved Institutional Review Board protocol.

3.1 Obtaining Surgical Biopsies of the Human Olfactory Mucosa

1. Surgical biopsies of olfactory mucosa can be collected in the operating room in patients undergoing endoscopic endonasal surgery under general anesthesia.

2. Apply 0.5% oxymetazoline spray in the nasal cavity for decongestion. *See* **Notes 1** and **2**.
3. Once the mucosa is decongested, examine the nasal cavity using 0 degree endoscope. Visualize the olfactory cleft mucosa along the superior nasal septum or the adjacent superior medial vertical lamella of the superior turbinate.
4. Be aware of the location of the cribriform plate, and avoid instrumentation of this area, as injury to the cribriform can cause a CSF leak.
5. At the selected biopsy site, sharply incise the mucosa approximately 1 cm with a #12 blade down to underlying bone.
6. Elevate the mucosa from the underlying bone using a cottle or a freer elevator. Avoid suctioning directly on the biopsy area, as this can de-epithelialize the biopsy tissue.
7. Excise the mucosa with a small straight through-cutting ethmoid forceps and place this onto saline-soaked Telfa gauze atraumatically.
8. Pass the Telfa/specimen off the field immediately and place into tube containing desired collection solution on ice. For transcriptomic assays, process immediately.

3.2 Nasal Cytology Brush Biopsies of the Human Olfactory Mucosa

1. If performing this procedure in the operating room under general anesthesia, follow **steps 1–3** in Subheading 3.1.
2. If performing this procedure on an awake subject, topical anesthetic spray (i.e., oxymetazoline with lidocaine or pontacaine) is applied to the olfactory cleft region, and the subject is reclined for about 10 minutes.
3. Once the mucosa is decongested, examine the nasal cavity using a 0 degree endoscope. Visualize the olfactory cleft mucosa along the superior nasal septum or the adjacent superior medial vertical lamella of the superior turbinate.
4. Advance the nasal cytology brush into the nasal cavity, and direct it to the olfactory cleft under direct endoscopic visualization (Fig. 2). Avoid excess contact with respiratory regions.
5. Rotate the brush two to three times gently to collect mucosal cells. Do this carefully to avoid traumatizing the mucosa and causing bleeding.
6. Place the brush into collection solution on ice. Move the brush repeatedly up and down in the buffer, to ensure cells are collected into the suspension.

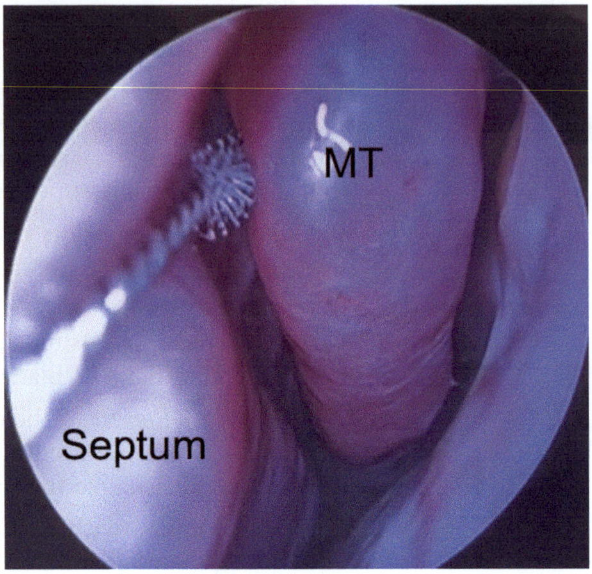

Fig. 2 Olfactory biopsy using nasal cytology brush. 0 degree nasal endoscopic view of the left nasal cavity. The cytology brush is positioned into the olfactory cleft, between the septum (labeled) and the middle turbinate (MT). Once advanced adequately, the brush is rotated to acquire surface epithelial cells

3.3 Tissue Processing for Frozen Section Immunohistochemistry

1. Obtain a piece of the surgical specimen and fix in 5 mL of desired fixative solution for 3 hours at room temperature. Aspirate or pour off the fixative into a designated waste bin.
2. Rinse the tissue in 5 mL of PBS three times for 5 min each time, and aspirate or pour off the supernatant.
3. Incubate the specimen in 5–15 ml cryoprotection/decalcification solution on a gentle rocker at 4° for 3–7 days.
4. Place the specimen into a small cryomold containing OCT medium.
5. Snap freeze the tissue on either dry ice powder or liquid nitrogen, and prepare cryosections immediately; alternatively block may be stored at −80° in a sealed tube (*see* **Note 5**).
6. Collect cryosections onto Superfrost Plus slides and store at −20° until use. If planning RNA in situ hybridization stains, store at −80°.

3.4 Sample Processing for Single-Cell Sequencing

1. Digest tissue or cells collected from cytology brush in 2.5 mL of enzyme cocktail 1 for 10–15 min at 37 °C. Triturate gently and frequently throughout the incubation period without making bubbles. The incubation period can be shorter for specimen collected by cytology brush. (Note: if a stringy precipitate is observed, this is extracellular DNA from dying cells; add up to 50 μl additional 1 mg/ml DNase solution.)

2. Add 2.5 mL of enzyme cocktail 2. Incubate for an additional 1–3 minutes 37 °C. Triturate several times.
3. Add 2.5 mL of FBS to deactivate enzymes.
4. If the sample was a surgical biopsy and any larger undigested tissue remains, add 5 ml HBSS and filter the sample through a 250 μm mesh strainer. Spin at 400 g × 5 min, resuspend in 500 μl of HBSS, and inspect/count cells.
5. Filter through a 70 μm mesh and centrifuge for 5 min at 400 g at 4 °C. Aspirate or pour off the supernatant.
6. *Optional.* If abundant red blood cells are observed in the pellet, resuspend in 3 ml ACK lysing buffer, and incubate at room temperature for 5 minutes with gentle rocking. Centrifuge for 5 minutes at 400 g at 4 °C, and aspirate or pour off the lysing buffer.
7. Wash samples in HBSS. Centrifuge for 5 minutes at 400 g at 4 ° C.
8. Resuspend in 300–500 μl of Resuspension solution, and adjust to a final concentration of one million cells/ml.

4 Notes

1. *Avoid* placing pledgets or packing into the nose, as this can debride the delicate mucosa, causing loss of surface epithelium from biopsy area.
2. Surgical-style biopsies may be obtained from awake patients in the clinic [14]. In this case, topical anesthetic spray (i.e., oxymetazoline with lidocaine or pontacaine) is applied to the olfactory cleft region, and the subject is reclined for about 10 min. Additional spray may be applied on a cotton pledget as needed to the middle turbinate just anterior to the olfactory cleft, but do not place the packing into the olfactory cleft region. Otherwise, the procedure is performed as described in Subheading 3.1. Any minor bleeding can be controlled with topical oxymetazoline. Significant obstruction due to septal deviation or anxiety preventing cooperation is contraindications to awake olfactory biopsy.
3. The olfactory cleft is located posterior to the middle turbinate heads, superiorly. With experience, it is possible to recognize subtle vascular stripes running inferior-superior in the olfactory cleft, representing the vessels of epineurium of the cranial nerve I fibers.
4. It is common for there to be patches of respiratory-like surface epithelium in the olfactory cleft [15, 16]. This is impossible to appreciate on endoscopic exam. It is more common in elderly

subjects and likely represents wear-and-tear or neurogenic exhaustion. It is more common in the most anterior region of the olfactory cleft.

5. When snap freezing fixed tissue specimens, avoid freezing artifact by treating at least 4 days in the cryoprotection solution, and freeze the tissue rapidly. We do this by dipping the bottom of the cryomold into liquid nitrogen for several seconds until at least half of the OCT has frozen, then immediately place into the cryostat. However, if the block is frozen too rapidly, it may fracture.
6. When handling human tissue specimens, use universal precautions, including the use of gloves or other personal protective equipment, in accordance with your institutional biosafety protocols.
7. Excess cells that are not loaded onto a 10X Chromium Controller can be frozen down to maintain viability for later assays, such as flow cytometry. Cells can be spun down to remove resuspension solution, then resuspended in 90% FBS, 10% DMSO in a cryo-vial. We recommend freezing cells slowly in an insulated chamber at −80°. Then cells can be stored long term in liquid nitrogen.
8. Olfactory biopsies may also be snap-frozen and stored for assays. For instance, snap-frozen samples stored under liquid nitrogen may be used for nuclear isolation for single-nucleus RNA-sequencing or ATAC-sequencing protocols. When snap freezing for other assays, we recommend proceeding with cell dissociation, as described above. At the final step, instead of resuspending the cell pellet in resuspension solution for 10X chromium loading, the pellet can be snap frozen with liquid nitrogen.

Acknowledgments

This work was support by NIH grants DC016859 and DC018371 (BJG).

References

1. Schwob JE et al (2017) Stem and progenitor cells of the mammalian olfactory epithelium: Taking poietic license. J Comp Neurol 525(4):1034–1054
2. Rawson NE et al (1997) Selectivity and response characteristics of human olfactory neurons. J Neurophysiol 77(3):1606–1613
3. Leopold DA et al (2000) Anterior distribution of human olfactory epithelium. Laryngoscope 110(3 Pt 1):417–421
4. Lane AP et al (2002) The superior turbinate as a source of functional human olfactory receptor neurons. Laryngoscope 112(7 Pt 1): 1183–1189

5. Doty RL (2015) Handbook of Olfaction and Gustation, 3rd edn. John Wiley & Sons, Incorporated
6. Choi R, Goldstein BJ (2018) Olfactory epithelium: Cells, clinical disorders, and insights from an adult stem cell niche. Laryngoscope Investig Otolaryngol 3(1):35–42
7. Holbrook EH et al (2011) Immunohistochemical characterization of human olfactory tissue. Laryngoscope 121(8):1687–1701
8. Holbrook EH, Leopold DA, Schwob JE (2005) Abnormalities of axon growth in human olfactory mucosa. Laryngoscope 115(12):2144–2154
9. Durante MA et al (2020) Single-cell analysis of olfactory neurogenesis and differentiation in adult humans. Nat Neurosci 23(3):323–326
10. Oliva AD et al (2022) Aging-related olfactory loss is associated with olfactory stem cell transcriptional alterations in humans. J Clin Invest
11. Finlay JB et al (2022) Persistent post-COVID-19 smell loss is associated with immune cell infiltration and altered gene expression in olfactory epithelium. Sci Transl Med 14(676): eadd0484
12. Orru CD et al (2014) A test for Creutzfeldt-Jakob disease using nasal brushings. N Engl J Med 371(6):519–529
13. Brozzetti L et al (2020) Neurodegeneration-Associated Proteins in Human Olfactory Neurons Collected by Nasal Brushing. Front Neurosci 14:145
14. Holbrook EH, Rebeiz L, Schwob JE (2016) Office-based olfactory mucosa biopsies. Int Forum Allergy Rhinol 6(6):646–653
15. Nakashima T, Kimmelman CP, Snow JB Jr (1984) Structure of human fetal and adult olfactory neuroepithelium. Arch Otolaryngol 110(10):641–646
16. Paik SI et al (1992) Human olfactory biopsy. The influence of age and receptor distribution. Arch Otolaryngol Head Neck Surg 118(7): 731–738

Chapter 11

Cranial Window for Acute and Chronic Optical Access to Record Neuronal Network Dynamics in the Olfactory Bulb

Marco Brondi and Claudia Lodovichi

Abstract

Cranial window implant is the preparation of choice for acute and chronic optical access to a given brain area. The cranial window provides a stable preparation, which can last for months. This window allows to follow the activity of distinct population of neurons expressing genetically encoded fluorescent reporters of activity in awake, behaving, head-fixed animals. The optical access can also be exploited for acute imaging, in anesthetized animals. Here we provide a detailed protocol for acute and chronic cranial window implantations in the olfactory bulb. We also provide the procedure to perform injections of adeno-associated viruses expressing genetically encoded fluorescent sensors in the same area.

Key words Olfactory bulb, Cranial window, AAVs, Fluorescent sensors

1 Introduction

Neuronal circuits in the central nervous system exhibit distinct patterns of activity both at rest and in response to stimuli [1–3]. The dynamics of this neuronal activity changes with time, according to the status of the experimental subject and the type of task performed. To understand the neuronal basis underlying a given behavior or a status, such as awake versus asleep, it is necessary to record the activity of a large population of neurons, with cellular resolution, in acute and for long period of time. The current availability of multiphoton imaging along with a large variety of genetically encoded fluorescent reporters of neuronal activity, such as calcium indicators [4], provide the suitable tools to analyze neuronal network dynamics. This unprecedented approach to brain activity has revolutionized our understanding of brain function. In particular, multiphoton calcium imaging represents a powerful technique and the most exploited approach to study the activity of a large population of neurons, with minimal invasiveness, in anesthetized and awake behaving animals.

Bradley J. Goldstein and Hiroaki Matsunami (eds.), *The Olfactory System*, Methods in Molecular Biology, vol. 2710, https://doi.org/10.1007/978-1-0716-3425-7_11,

However, it is often difficult to focus light on the animal brain through the intact skull and collect high-quality and high-resolution imaging, owing to light scattering caused by the bone. To overcome these limitations and gain optical access to the brain, it is convenient to create a "window" into the skull. This procedure is critical and essential for a high-quality two-photon imaging. Transgenic lines of mice expressing CRE recombinase, suitable for driving the expression of calcium indicators in reporter mouse lines are available [5]. However, adeno-associated viral (AAV) vectors expressing genetically encoded calcium sensors still offer higher degrees of flexibility in terms of experimental designs.

Furthermore, the calcium reporter construct is continuously engineered to optimize its performance, making the viral vector a unique useful tool to deliver the most recent version of genetically encoded sensor to the neuronal population [6–8].

Several protocols are available for acute and/or chronic window preparation in different brain regions [9–13]. Very few, however, have addressed the procedure for cranial window implant in the olfactory bulb, although this brain region has been the center of a growing number of studies [14–22]. Here, we provide a detailed protocol for acute and chronic cranial window implants in the olfactory bulb. We also provide a detailed procedure to perform AAV injections in the same brain area.

Although fluorescent calcium indicators are widely used to record neuronal activity, a large variety of genetically encoded fluorescent sensors for neurotransmitters and neuromodulators are currently available [23–26]. The procedures here described can be applied to any of the available indicators.

2 Materials

2.1 Animals

Wild-type mice (C57BL/6); (both sexes, 4–12 weeks old, average weight 20–30 g at the time of surgery). Any procedure must be conducted in accordance with institutional and national guidelines and regulations.

2.2 Solutions and Drugs

1. Ketamine-xylazine injectable solution. Ketamine 100–200 mg/Kg body weight (50 mg/mL) and xylazine 5–16 mg/Kg (20 mg/mL), diluted in isotonic physiological solution (0.9% mass/volume NaCl).
2. Lidocaine injectable solution 2.5 mM, topic or subcutaneous administration.
3. Iodopovidone 10%, topic administration.
4. Hydrogen peroxide 3.6%.

5. Dexamethasone sodium phosphate 2 mg/Kg body weight, typically 100 μL of 0.4 mg/mL in isotonic physiological solution, administered by intramuscular injection.
6. Tramadol chlorhydrate 25 mg/Kg body weight, administered by intraperitoneal injection.
7. Enrofloxacin, 85 mg/Kg/day in drinking water.
8. Lacrigel, topic administration.
9. Artificial cerebrospinal fluid (ACSF, sterile): 119 mM $NaCl_2$, 6.2 mM $NaHCO_3$, 2.5 mM KCl, 1 mM NaH_2PO_4, 1.3 mM $MgCl_2$, 10 mM glucose. Gas with 5% CO_2/95%.
   (a) O_2 for 10–15 min, then add 2.5 mM $CaCl_2$. Filter sterilize with a 0.22 μm filter apparatus, and store at 4 °C. ACSF is stable for 3–4 weeks.
10. Ethanol 70%.
11. Adeno-associated viruses (AAV) expressing the fluorescent reporter of neuronal activity such as GCaMP (https://www.addgene.org/). Carefully choose serotype and promoter during the experimental planning. In our hands AAV2.1 or 2.9 with CAG or hSyn promoters provide an efficient labelling, staining mitral and tufted cells along with periglomerular and juxtaglomerular cells.
12. Isoflurane along with its delivery apparatus (chronic imaging) (https://www.harvardapparatus.com/tabletop-anesthesia-systems.html).

2.3 Equipment

1. Stereotaxic apparatus (https://stoeltingco.com/Neuroscience/New-Standardtm-Stereotaxic-Instruments-for-Rats-and-Mice~9650).
2. A wide stainless surgical surface to arrange all the surgical tools and other items related to the surgery.
3. Magnetic-based stand, select a bulky one for stability (https://www.thorlabs.com/).
4. Manual or digital three axes linear stage micromanipulator attached to the stand (https://www.newport.com/c/manual-linear-stages, https://stoeltingco.com/Neuroscience/New-Standardtm-Stereotaxic-Instruments-for-Rats-and-Mice~9650). Allow ~10–20 cm excursion in the vertical axis to ease the placement of the microinjection syringe pump apparatus.
5. Stereo microscope (1–6 X objective) with long working distance (30–60 cm). The presence of the fluorescence module is desirable but not strictly necessary.

6. Illumination system with optic fibers (https://www.wpiinc.com/var-3776-high- intensity-fiber-optic-illumination-source).
7. Head-holding bars + head-plates (usually custom made).
8. Running wheel, easily done with a 3D printer (chronic imaging).
9. Optical glue (chronic imaging) (https://www.norlandprod.com/adhesives/noa%2071.html).
10. UV lamp.
11. Low melting agarose (optional).
12. PDMS + curing agent 10:1 (optional) (SYLGARD https://www.dow.com/en- us/pdp.sylgard-184-silicone-elastomer-kit.01064291z.html).
13. Microinjection syringe pump with nL precision (e.g., https://www.wpi-europe.com/products/pumps-and-microinjection/micro-syringe-pump%2D%2Dstereotaxic-injection/ump3-3.aspx).
14. Hamilton syringe, 10 μL, (700 series).
15. Micropipette puller.
16. Borosilicate glass capillaries (standard, single barrel) 100 mm long, outer diameter: 2 mm, inner diameter: 1.12 mm (e.g., https://www.sutter.com for pulling procedures).
17. Mineral oil.
18. Micromotor drill (up to 38,000 rpm, e.g., https://stoeltingco.com/Neuroscience/Micromotor-Drill~9753).
19. Drill burrs (steel, round, no point 0.3–0.4 mm https://www.busch.eu/en/).
20. Syringes (28 and 15 gauge).
21. Round glass coverslips, 5 mm and 3 mm in diameter (mostly chronic imaging 0.15 mm thick).
22. Superbond universal kit dental cement (chronic imaging) (e.g., https://www.dentaltrey.it/superbond-universal-kit-k058e.html).
23. Homeothermic blanket.

Animal subjects:

Wild-type mice (C57BL/6); (Jackson Laboratories, both sexes, 4–12 weeks old, average weight 2030 g at the time of surgery). Any procedure must be conducted in accordance with institutional and national guidelines and regulations.

2.4 Surgical Instruments and Various Items

1. Small curved scissors.
2. Straight and curved tweezers (2 x type).
3. Razor blades.
4. Animal hair trimmer.
5. Surgifoam (e.g., https://www.jnjmedtech.com/en-US/product/ethicon-surgifoam-absorbable-gelatin-sponge),
6. Cyanoacrylate/Loctite 401.
7. Kimwipes.
8. Biological waste container.
9. Vials (1–2 mL), falcon tubes (15–50 mL).
10. Pipettes (P200, P20, P2) and relative tips.
11. Parafilm.
12. Plastic box (e.g., an empty pipette tip box).
13. Permanent marker with thin tip.
14. Glass beads sterilizer.

3 Methods

3.1 Procedures for Injecting AAV Expressing Genetically Encoded Sensors into the Olfactory Bulb

1. Setting: Pull borosilicate glass capillaries with thin and long shaft (about 3 mm in length) to minimize tissue damage during the glass pipette penetration in the brain parenchyma. The glass pipette can be shaped with open or closed tips. If you opt for open tips, make sure the opening is around 10um in diameter, in the second case, see point 8, optional.
2. Clean the whole surgical surface and the stereotaxic apparatus with an antiseptic, and let them dry. Sterilize all surgical tools with antiseptic solution or in a hot glass bead sterilizer.
3. Wrap the heating pad with a thin paper, and place the thermocouple probe in contact with the heating pad and the mouse abdomen. This configuration allows to keep constant the temperature of the blanket and in turn the mouse body temperature. Turn on the thermostatic system and set it to 37 °C.
4. Set the focus of the stereomicroscope on the animal head and allow for enough room for focus adjustments (i.e., set the microscope around half of the maximal excursion in all available axis).
5. Place the microinjection syringe pump on the stand, above the stereotaxic apparatus, in a position that allows for approximately 40–60 cm excursion in the vertical axis and 10–20 cm excursion along the horizontal plane.

6. Place the optical fibers for optimal illumination of the surgical field.
7. Place the drill and the microinjection pump controller in close proximity to the surgical field.
8. Set the microinjection syringe pump controller to the desired volume to be injected. If the tip of the glass capillaries is closed (see point 1), break the tip gently scraping it on a piece of paper or Kimwipe or using tweezers (pay attention to break a very small portion of the tip). Remove the air-tight lock and the plunger from the Hamilton syringe. Pay attention to keep all the small parts in order to be able to reassemble the syringe properly.
9. Fill the barrel of the Hamilton syringe with mineral oil, using a15 gauge syringe. Avoid air bubbles formation during the filling. Fill with additional mineral oil the Hamilton syringe from the needle side to reduce the risk of air bubbles formation in the following steps. Insert again the air-tight lock components in the Hamilton syringe, but do not tighten it, to allow the insertion of the glass borosilicate capillary.
10. Gently insert the filled capillary in the air-tight lock system of the Hamilton syringe, and then tighten it. The capillary must be aligned with the rest of the Hamilton syringe. Misalignments prevent a proper use of the syringe and compromise the AAV injection. Insert the plunger in the Hamilton syringe, and slowly press it in, to eject part of the oil and make room for the AAV solution. In our experience, if less than a total volume of 5 μL has to be injected (for several animals), we suggest to eject half the oil volume from the Hamilton syringe in order to operate with half the available range. Inspect for the presence of air bubbles along the barrel of Hamilton syringe and along the capillary. Proceed only if air bubbles are absent, otherwise dispose of the capillary and start again.
11. Place the Hamilton syringe with the glass pipette in the syringe housing on the microinjection syringe pump system. Place an empty small box (i.e., an empty tip box) covered with a piece of firmly stretched parafilm under the tip of the glass capillary.
12. Prepare the desired dilution of the AAV (suggested 1:1–1:2). Always keep the AAV vials on ice. Put at least 4 μL of diluted AAV on the parafilm. Consider 500 nL per injection site and set the AAV volume to load in the capillary accordingly.
13. Lower the tip of the glass pipette into the AAV solution drop, avoiding any contacts with the parafilm, to prevent tip breakage. Perform this procedure under the stereomicroscope (2–3 X) to control the tip position.

14. Set the microinjection syringe pump controller on the withdrawal mode, 1 μL/min rate and withdraw the AAV solution drop. Each withdrawal step will uptake 1 μL of solution, thus repeat withdrawal steps until complete collection of the drop.

3.2 Surgical Procedures for Viral Injections

1. Weigh the animal.
2. Anesthetize the mouse with an intraperitoneal (i.p.) injection of ketamine (0.10 mg/g body weight) and xylazine (0.01 mg/g body weight). Alternatively, 1.25% avertin (0.02 mL/g body weight) or isoflurane (4% for induction; 1.5–2% for surgery in 0.5 L/min O_2). Higher susceptibility to dura bleeding during surgery under isoflurane anesthesia has been observed.

   After ketamine/xylazine or avertin injection, place the animal in the cage, under a heating lamp to maintain body temperature, and wait till the mouse is deeply anesthetized (usually 10–20 min). If the anesthetic of choice is isoflurane, gently place the mouse in an anesthesia induction chamber, and induce deep anesthesia with 3% isoflurane. Note: anesthesia should induce within 2 min.
3. Once the animal is deeply anesthetized, gently transfer the mouse in the stereotaxic apparatus equipped with the heating blanket set on 37 °C. Stabilize the head with blunt ear bars, and, in case of isoflurane anesthesia, put the isoflurane mask on the nose of the animal. Be sure that the nose clamp of the stereotaxic apparatus does not reach the nasal aspect of the eyes.
4. Check reflexes (tail pinch and/or eyelid reflex).

   If the animal is still awake or lightly anesthetized, consider waiting another 10 min, and then check again the reflexes (point 27). If after 40 min the animal is not properly anesthetized, inject another 100–200 μL of anesthetic. In case of isoflurane anesthesia, increase the isoflurane flow up to 1–2 L/min until the animal is deeply anesthetized, usually within 2 min, and reduced the anesthetic flow to 0.5 L/ min to maintain a constant level of the anesthesia. Check the reflex again (point 27), and when properly anesthetized, place the mouse in the stereotaxic (see point 26).
5. Shave the head of the animal using a veterinary hair clipper. Use a blade specific for small animal with fine hair. Alternatively, use hair removal cream. Leave the cream on the head for 5–10 min (follow the instructions of the cream), and then clean it off. For a thorough air removal, the two procedures can be combined: first use the veterinary hair clipper and then apply the hair removal cream. Pay attention to keep the hair removal cream away from the animal eyes. The hair removal cream can irritate

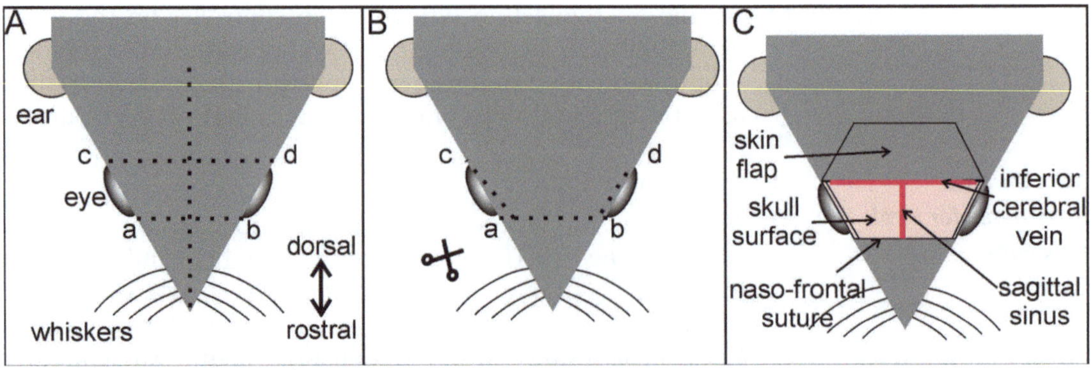

Fig. 1 Schematic of the surgery to expose the skull overlying the olfactory bulb. (**a**) schematic of the dorsal view of the mouse head. The vertical dotted line indicates the midline, while the horizontal dotted lines represent the rostral (indicated by the dotted line between a and b) and caudal (indicated by the dotted line between c–d) aspects of the eyes. (**b**) Dotted lines indicate the cuts: a–b, horizontal incision; a–c; and b–d, the diagonal cuts. (**c**) The skin flap is placed over the posterior region of the head, exposing the skull overlying the bulb. This area extends from the inferior cerebral vein to the nasofrontal suture. The sagittal sinus can be easily seen along the midline

the skin if applied for long period of time, therefore follow the instructions carefully. Avoid excessive usage of hair removal cream. Wash off the residuals of the cream and the hair, using iodine or ethanol 70%. This procedure provides local and immediate disinfection of the surface.

6. Wipe the scalp with cotton swabs soaked in iodopovidone. Apply abundant ophthalmic ointment (such as Lacrigel) on both eyes to prevent dehydration and irritation, and provide some physical protection.
7. Apply lidocaine solution on the scalp and wait 3–5 min for induction of local anesthesia. Before starting the surgery, sterilize all the instruments with antiseptic solution or in a glass bead sterilizer. Cut horizontally the scalp at the level of the line connecting the rostral aspect of the eyes (see Fig. 1b). Use this incision to make two additional cuts along the diagonal line connecting the lateral edges of the incision and the caudal aspect of the eyes (see Fig. 1b).
8. Put the skin flap over the posterior side of the head (see Fig. 1c).
9. Wipe the skull with cotton swabs soaked in hydrogen peroxide. Allow the hydrogen peroxide to act for few seconds. Wipe off the excess of hydrogen peroxide. Keep the hydrogen peroxide away from the eyes of the mouse. Apply lidocaine on the skull.
10. Remove the periosteum gently scraping the skull with a scalpel blade or tweezers. Wash the skull with physiological solution; can be repeated to completely eliminate connective tissue and periosteum.

11. Apply a few drops of physiological solution on the skull and wipe off the excess. This cleaning procedure makes visible bregma, the inferior cerebral vein and the nasal portion of the sagittal sinus (Fig. 1c).

3.3 AAV Injections

1. Align the capillary tip to bregma, using the micromanipulator. Then move the pipette to the area of the olfactory bulb to be injected, using bregma as reference point. We generally use the following coordinate with respect to bregma: anterior, 4.5 mm; lateral, 0.8 mm, in each olfactory bulb. Keep the tip of the capillary in proximity of the skull to avoid parallax, being careful not to break the tip against the skull.
2. Once reached the area to be injected, move up the capillary along the vertical axis and sign on the skull the injection site with a fine tip permanent marker. Perform this procedure on each olfactory bulb.
3. Wipe the skull with cotton swabs soaked in iodopovidone. Keep iodine away from the eyes of the mouse, and avoid excessive usage of iodine.
4. Make a small hole (about 0.5 mm in diameter) on the marked spot on the skull of each olfactory bulb, using a burr of 0.3 mm diameter, and a low-medium drill speed. Do not drill deep to avoid touching the dura mater.
5. Wipe the skull surface with sterile ACSF.
6. Set the coordinates of the small hole (Subheading 3.3 **step 1**) on the micromanipulator.
7. Slowly move the capillary downward, perforate the meninges, and reach a depth of 400–500 um. If any bleeding occurs, stop immediately, and pull the capillary out of the brain parenchyma. Wipe the area with cotton swabs soaked in sterile ACSF. Wait for the bleeding to stop and start again from point 50. Keep away from the first penetration, which caused the bleeding. If subsequent attempts end up in further bleeding, consider the following:
   (a) Drill another hole in a nearby location, and repeat the procedure from (Subheading 3.3 **step 1**).
   (b) Forgo injecting this bulb if a significant bleeding persists.
   (c) If the bleeding is negligible, you may consider to proceed.
8. Set the microinjection syringe pump controller to "injection mode" with the following settings: 500 nL total volume to be injected, 70 nL/min injection rate.
9. Start the injection. Check for bleeding or solution spillover during the injection. Some cerebrospinal fluid spill is expected in the first seconds. If bleeding or abundant cerebrospinal fluid

spillover is observed, consider alternative approaches described in point 50.

10. Once the injection is completed, keep the capillary in place for at least 2 min, then withdraw the capillary.
11. Move the capillary slowly (1 min approximately) till out of the parenchyma. Then, place the capillary away from the injected area, using the micromanipulator. Wipe the injected area with sterile ACSF and remove the excess.
12. Repeat the procedure to inject the other olfactory bulb.
13. Once completed the second injection, apply a few drops of sterile ACSF on the skull to clean the surface.
14. Place the skin flap back on the skull and apply a small drop of cyanoacrylate along the edges to seal the skin flap with the sculp. Keep the cyanoacrylate away from the eyes of the mouse. Avoid or at least minimize the spillover of the cyanoacrylate along the margins. Wait about 10 min to let the glue dry.
15. Remove the animal from the stereotaxic apparatus.
16. Administer dexamethasone sodium phosphate (~2 ug/body weight) and Tramadol Chlorhydrate (25 mg/Kg body weight) by intramuscular injection in the quadriceps muscle. Dexamethasone reduces cortical stress response during the surgery and prevents brain edema.
17. House the animal in its cage, under a warming lamp till complete recovery from the anesthesia. Once the mouse is fully awake and behaving, house it back in the animal house.

After some practice, the whole procedure should be performed in about 30 min.

GCaMP expression peaks at ~2–3 weeks after the injection and remains stable for at least one month.

3.4 Procedures for Cranial Window Implantation for Acute Imaging in Anesthetized Mice

After 2 weeks from the injection, it is possible to perform the surgical procedure to create a cranial window for imaging, as described in the following steps:

1. Anesthetize the mouse (see above) and follow the initial procedure described in Subheading 3.1.
2. Cut the skin along the midline to expose the skull above the olfactory bulb. In cutting the skin along the lateral aspects of the olfactory bulb, be very careful not to damage the eyelids or the eye. This will cause profuse bleeding, making necessary to sacrifice the mouse. Do not cut away the skin, as it will be used as a wall around the craniotomy, to retain the water into the craniotomy.
3. Draw with a permanent marker or engrave with 0.5 diameter drill bit, a circle about 3 mm in diameter on the skull above

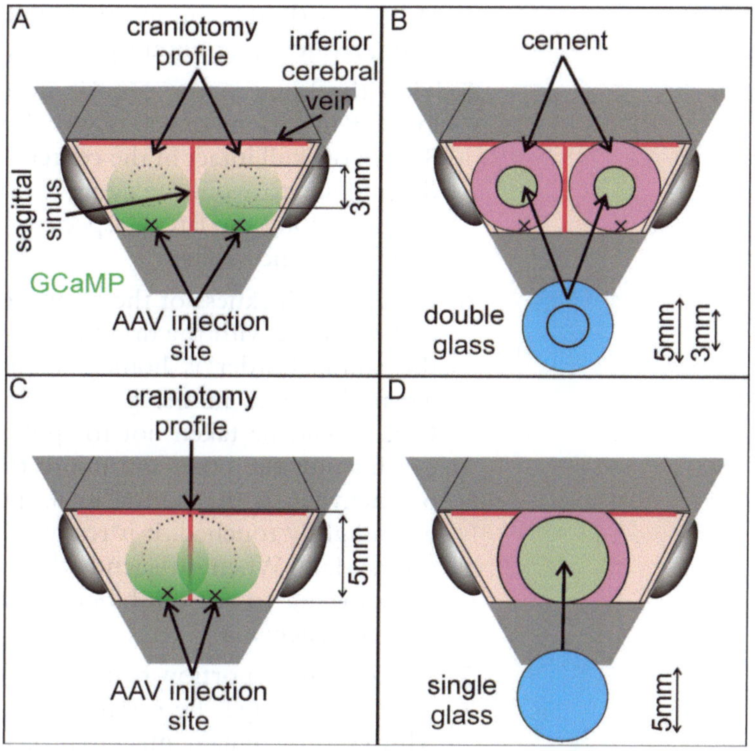

Fig. 2 Window surgery. (**a**) Schematic of the 3 mm diameter craniotomy on the skull above each olfactory bulb (OB). The perimeter of the craniotomy should be far from the inferior cerebral vein and the sagittal sinus. (**b**) Chronic window implantation. A double glass, 3 mm in diameter (green) and 5 mm in diameter (purple) are placed in the craniotomy and sealed to the skull by the cement. (**c**) Schematic of the 5 mm craniotomy on the skull overlying both OB. (**d**) A double glass is placed in the craniotomy and sealed to the skull

each bulb. The circle extends from the inferior cerebral vein to the nasofrontal suture, centered on the midline. Alternatively, draw a bigger circle (about 5 mm in diameter) including both olfactory bulbs. The latter procedure is more challenging, since the sagittal sinus is located along the midline, separating the two olfactory bulbs (Fig. 2a, c).

4. Thin the bone around the marked circles/engraving. Drill with smooth and homogeneous motion, maintaining a shallow angle between the drill bit and the skull. While drilling, apply minimal pressure on the skull, to avoid cracking the bone and damage the brain parenchyma. Interrupt drilling with frequent pauses and wash the skull with ice-cold ACSF or saline, to clean and cool down the bone. These pauses are essential, as drilling for too long in the same location causes over heating the skull and damage the dura, blood vessels, and brain parenchyma.

Drilling without caution causes inflammation/damage in the brain, reducing significantly 2P imaging quality.

5. Thin the bone in the circular groove around the region of interest in a homogeneous way, leaving a portion (diameter 3 mm) of skull intact in the center. Drill carefully and far from the midline, to avoid damaging the superior sagittal sinus. Drill carefully along the lateral aspects of the olfactory bulb, as it is adjacent to the orbits.
6. Check the thickness of the bone along the groove applying a light pressure with the drill tip or tweezers, and ascertain that the whole border is homogeneously thinned. Stop drilling when the bone in the groove can be easily pushed down. Care should be taken not to apply excessive pressure, as this can fracture the bone and injure the dura and eventually the parenchyma. If the central intact portion of the bone moves when lightly touched, it is ready to be removed. Apply ACSF on the skull. When sufficiently thin, the bone appears transparent allowing to see the blood vasculature in the underneath brain parenchyma.
7. Pierce a small portion of the thinned bone using the tip of 28 gauge syringe. Be careful not to damage the dura mater, which should remain intact to protect the brain and favor high-quality imaging. Attempts of dura removal can easily results in bleeding and damage of the superficial brain layer.
8. Carefully proceed in fracturing the thinned bone in the groove. Note: some bleeding is expected from the skull, due to the tearing of the vasculature plexus in the trabecular section of the cranial bone. Once the whole perimeter is fractured, use the syringe tip or tweezers to lift and remove the bone patch overlying the olfactory bulb.
9. Apply ACSF to the exposed brain surface, and wipe off the excess without touching the brain surface. Under ideal circumstances the dura should remain intact with no bleeding. However, as the dura is attached to the bone, some superficial blood vessels, i.e., capillaries, might bleed. Small focal bleedings tend to resolve spontaneously or can be controlled by applying GELfoam or washing the surface with ACSF. If abundant bleeding occurs, the animal has to be sacrificed. The brain surface exposed is now clean and the vasculature on the surface of the brain clearly visible and intact.
10. (optional) To reduce motion artifacts due to heartbeat, a glass coverslip can be placed in the craniotomy filled with a drop of low melting point agarose (4%). Agarose must be below 37 °C yet still fluid when applied. Once the agarose has solidified, trim the excess from the surface of the bone around the craniotomy, using a scalpel. Place the 5 mm coverslip on top of the

agarose and aided by a syringe tip, drop cyanoacrylate along the edge of the glass coverslip, to glue the coverslip to the skull. Wait to get the glue dry. Care should be taken to control the temperature of the agarose: if too hot, it could damage the brain; if too solid, it can't flow into the craniotomy. Be careful not to spill cyanoacrylate on the brain parenchyma, as it causes damage. In our experience, this step can be skipped if the surgery is performed in the proper way and the animal is in stable metabolic conditions, as motion artifacts are negligible.

11. (optional) A drop of PDMS (in the proportion 10:1 PDMS/curing agent) can be used instead of agarose and glass coverslip (point 15). Polymer and curing agent have to be prepared in advance (30 min ahead of the whole procedure). PDMS will be then applied to fill the craniotomy and gently cover the surrounding bone. Leave some bone uncovered in order to use cyanoacrylate to glue the PDMS to the skull. Wait 10–15 min to let the PDMS dry.
12. During the surgical procedure, keep the animal hydrated by injecting a small amount of saline under the skin of the mouse with an insulin syringe (i.e., 1 mL syringe with a very fine needle). This procedure should be repeated during the imaging session (see below), especially if it lasts for several hours.
13. The cranial window is now completed. Maintain the animal in the stereotaxic frame equipped with the heating pad, and transfer the mouse to the two-photon microscope setup.
14. Place the isoflurane nose mask on the snout of the mouse to maintain the anesthesia level. Set isoflurane flux at 0.5–1% with 0.5 L/min O_2 with 1 bar air pressure. The level of anesthesia can be modulated during the imaging experiment, changing the percentage of isoflurane flux. Care should be taken to maintain constant the mouse body temperature.

3.5 Procedures for Chronic Cranial Window Implantation for Chronic Imaging

This procedure aims to combine the AAV viral injection and the placement of a chronic optical window on the olfactory bulbs in a single surgical session, in order to reduce animal stress and increase the success rate of the procedure.

1. Prepare a "double coverslip" (more than one couple is suggested) ahead of the surgical procedure. The double cover slip is formed by two coverslips, one of 3 and one of 5 mm in diameter. Place one coverslip on top of the other in a concentric manner. Seal the two coverslips adding a drop of optical glue between the two coverslips. Do not spill the glue outside the edges of the smaller coverslip.
2. The coverslips must then be placed under a UV lamp for 30–60 min to let the glue dry.

3. Follow the steps described in Subheading 3.1.
4. Mark/engrave (see point 68) a circle 3 mm in diameter on the skull overlying each olfactory bulb (Fig. 2a). Alternatively mark/engrave a circle of 5 mm, around both olfactory bulbs, and centered on the midline (Fig. 2c). Stay 1–2 mm away from the rostral rhinal vein, to avoid drilling on the skull above the vein, as it would easily cause a profuse bleeding. In the latter case, sacrifice the animal.
5. Proceed as described in Subheading 3.4, **Steps 4–9**.
6. Follow the steps described in Subheading 3.3, **Steps 1–13**.
7. Sterilize the double coverslips with ethanol 70%, wait for the ethanol to evaporate, then rinse the coverslips in sterilized ACSF.

Wash the brain surface with ACSF and then place the double coverslips, with the 3 mm glass facing the brain surface, in the craniotomy (Fig. 2b). In case of a single craniotomy, apply a 5 mm glass on the brain surface (Fig. 2d). Apply a gentle pressure to fit it in place. The glass coverslip should be as close to the brain as possible (~100um).

8. The surface of the skull should be dried again. Then apply a few drops of cyanoacrylate along the edge of the 5 mm glass coverslip and on the dried skull. Care should be taken to avoid any contact of the cyanoacrylate with the dura, as it will not remain transparent, making impossible to perform imaging.
9. Allow for the glue to dry.
10. Prepare the Superbond dental cement, (following the instructions), in the provided ceramic well, and placed it on ice to retard solidification.
11. Seal the perimeter of the 5 mm coverslip to the surrounding bone with the cement (Fig. 2b, d).
12. Wait until the cement dry. The cranial window is now completed. During the surgery care should be taken to maintain the mouse hydrated (see point 79).

In the following steps, we will describe the procedure to add the head post, required to fix the mouse head during the imaging session.

13. Remove the dorsal skin flap to expose the occipital portion of the skull (Fig. 3).
14. Clean the surface of the skull with ACSF and hydrogen peroxide. Add local lidocaine (4%), and wait a few minutes for the induction of local anesthesia.
15. Gently scrape the skull to remove the periosteum and the connective tissue.

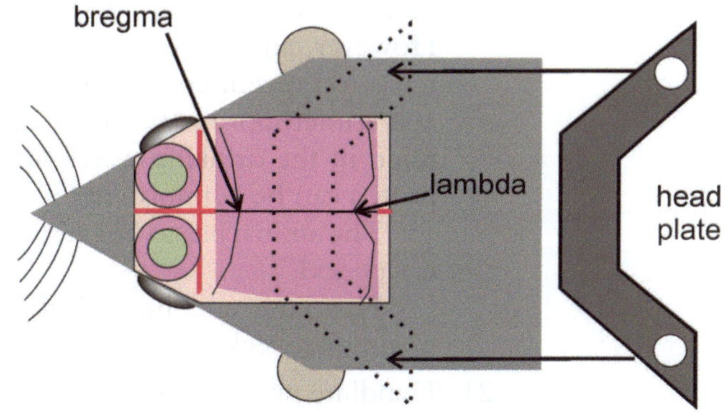

Fig. 3 Head-plate implant. Schematic of the dorsal aspect of the mouse head. The skull from about lambda to bregma is exposed (dark purple rectangle). Make sure to expose a large cranial surface to cement the metal bar to the bone

16. Engrave the surface of the skull exposed to create a rough surface. This creates a stronger adhesion of the glue to the skull where the head post has to be fix.
17. Sterilize the metal post for head fixation with ethanol 70%. Allow for the ethanol to evaporate, and then rinse the head post with sterile ACSF.
18. Apply a few drops of cyanoacrylate underneath the metal bar, and place it on the occipital bone without any overlap with the cement surrounding the cranial window (Fig. 3). Wait for the glue to dry.
19. Prepare Superbond dental cement. Apply the cement on the perimeter of the metal bar and on its dorsal surface in order to secure it to the skull (Fig. 3). Care should be taken to cover the entire head post base, to guarantee stability. Do not add too much cement as this cement wall might hamper objective movement and placement.
20. For chronic experiments lactated ringer solution (i.p. or s.c. 0.015 mL/g body weight; saline is also sufficient), and the antibiotic enrofloxacin (optional; s.c. 5 ug/g body weight) may be administered to prevent dehydration and infection, respectively. Allow the animal to recover on the heating pad and then under the warming lamp, and return it to its cage. Wet food is preferred in this period, to facilitate chewing and hydration. To alleviate pain, analgesic such as buprenorphine (Buprenex s.c. 0.1 ug/g body weight, twice per day) may be administered for 2–5 days. Allow the mouse to recover for additional 7–10 days. The cranial window usually improves during this recovery period. Large cages with high ceilings have to be preferred as they can help mice from damaging the window or detaching the head post. The cranial window can

remain clear for months without additional interventions. However, antibiotics and anti-inflammatory may be administered to prevent complications; sulfamethoxazole (1 mg/mL) and trimethoprim (0.2 mg/mL) can be chronically administered in the drinking water throughout the experiment. Carprofen can be administered daily i.p. or s.c.

The animal has to be carefully monitored during this recovery period.

Handling and head fixation habituation procedures can begin one week after the surgery.

21. Handling procedures: for the first 1–2 days the animal has to be gently handled by the experimenter, allowing it to voluntarily climb on the hand, rest in the palm as long as desired, and eat some food pellet from the hand palm.
22. Start the head fixation habituation, after 3 days.
23. The animal is fixed to the head fixation post, and then it is placed on the running wheel. Initially the mouse walks on the running wheel for 1–2 min. In the following days, the mouse stays on the running wheel for increasingly longer amount of time till reaching a period of about 60–120 min, after about 7 days of training.
24. The animal will always have free access to water during the training.
25. If the animal freely runs on the wheel by this time and shows no signs of stress, the imaging sessions can be started at the end of the second week after the chronic window implantation.
26. Additional time will be required in case the animal has to be trained for a particular behavioral task.

References

1. Augustinaite S, Kuhn B (2020) Complementary Ca2+ Activity of Sensory Activated and Suppressed Layer 6 Corticothalamic Neurons Reflects Behavioral State. Curr Biol 30:3945–3960.e5. https://doi.org/10.1016/j.cub.2020.07.069
2. Chen T-W, Wardill TJ, Sun Y, Pulver SR, Renninger SL, Baohan A, Schreiter ER, Kerr RA, Orger MB, Jayaraman V, Looger LL, Svoboda K, Kim DS (2013) Ultrasensitive fluorescent proteins for imaging neuronal activity. Nature 499:295–300. https://doi.org/10.1038/nature12354
3. Yang W, Yuste R (2017) In vivo imaging of neural activity. Nat Methods 14:349–359. https://doi.org/10.1038/nmeth.4230
4. Broussard GJ, Liang R, Tian L (2014) Monitoring activity in neural circuits with genetically encoded indicators. Front Mol Neurosci 7:97. https://doi.org/10.3389/fnmol.2014.00097
5. Madisen L, Garner AR, Shimaoka D, Chuong AS, Klapoetke NC, Li L, van der Bourg A, Niino Y, Egolf L, Monetti C, Gu H, Mills M, Cheng A, Tasic B, Nguyen TN, Sunkin SM, Benucci A, Nagy A, Miyawaki A, Helmchen F, Empson RM, Knöpfel T, Boyden ES, Reid RC, Carandini M, Zeng H (2015) Transgenic mice for intersectional targeting of neural sensors and effectors with high specificity and performance. Neuron 85:942–958. https://doi.org/10.1016/j.neuron.2015.02.022
6. Goertsen D, Flytzanis NC, Goeden N, Chuapoco MR, Cummins A, Chen Y, Fan Y,

Zhang Q, Sharma J, Duan Y, Wang L, Feng G, Chen Y, Ip NY, Pickel J, Gradinaru V (2022) AAV capsid variants with brain-wide transgene expression and decreased liver targeting after intravenous delivery in mouse and marmoset. Nat Neurosci 25:106–115. https://doi.org/10.1038/s41593-021-00969-4

7. Maturana CJ, Verpeut JL, Kooshkbaghi M, Engel EA (2021) Novel tool to quantify with single-cell resolution the number of incoming AAV genomes co- expressed in the mouse nervous system. Gene Ther. https://doi.org/10.1038/s41434-021-00272-8
8. Nectow AR, Nestler EJ (2020) Viral tools for neuroscience. Nat Rev Neurosci 21:669–681. https://doi.org/10.1038/s41583-020-00382-z
9. Carandini M, Shimaoka D, Rossi LF, Sato TK, Benucci A, Knöpfel T (2015) Imaging the awake visual cortex with a genetically encoded voltage indicator. J Neurosci 35:53–63. https://doi.org/10.1523/JNEUROSCI.0594-14.2015
10. Couto J, Musall S, Sun XR, Khanal A, Gluf S, Saxena S, Kinsella I, Abe T, Cunningham JP, Paninski L, Churchland AK (2021) Chronic, cortex-wide imaging of specific cell populations during behavior. Nat Protoc 16:3241–3263. https://doi.org/10.1038/s41596-021-00527-z
11. Heo C, Park H, Kim Y-T, Baeg E, Kim YH, Kim S-G, Suh M (2016) A soft, transparent, freely accessible cranial window for chronic imaging and electrophysiology. Sci Rep 6: 27818. https://doi.org/10.1038/srep27818
12. Low RJ, Gu Y, Tank DW (2014) Cellular resolution optical access to brain regions in fissures: Imaging medial prefrontal cortex and grid cells in entorhinal cortex. Proc Natl Acad Sci 111: 18739–18744. https://doi.org/10.1073/pnas.1421753111
13. Steinzeig A, Molotkov D, Castrén E (2017) Chronic imaging through "transparent skull" in mice. PLoS One 12:e0181788. https://doi.org/10.1371/journal.pone.0181788
14. Attems J, Walker L, Jellinger KA (2014) Olfactory bulb involvement in neurodegenerative diseases. Acta Neuropathol 127:459–475. https://doi.org/10.1007/s00401-014-1261-7
15. Bhattarai JP, Etyemez S, Jaaro-Peled H, Janke E, Leon Tolosa UD, Kamiya A, Gottfried JA, Sawa A, Ma M (2022) Olfactory modulation of the medial prefrontal cortex circuitry: Implications for social cognition. Seminars in Cell & Developmental Biology, Special Issue: Molecular dissection of cognition, emotion and thought by Akira Sawa & Takeshi Sakurai/Special Issue: Emerging biology of cellular protrusions in 3D architecture by Mayu Inaba and Mark Terasaki 129:31–39. https://doi.org/10.1016/j.semcdb.2021.03.022
16. Doty RL (2012) Olfaction in Parkinson's disease and related disorders. Neurobiol Dis 46: 527–552. https://doi.org/10.1016/j.nbd.2011.10.026
17. Gill JV, Lerman GM, Zhao H, Stetler BJ, Rinberg D, Shoham S (2020) Precise holographic manipulation of olfactory circuits reveals coding features determining perceptual detection. Neuron 108:382–393.e5. https://doi.org/10.1016/j.neuron.2020.07.034
18. Kudryavitskaya E, Marom E, Shani-Narkiss H, Pash D, Mizrahi A (2021) Flexible categorization in the mouse olfactory bulb. Curr Biol 31: 1616–1631.e4. https://doi.org/10.1016/j.cub.2021.01.063
19. Maset A, Albanesi M, di Soccio A, Canova M, Dal Maschio M, Lodovichi C (2021) Aberrant patterns of sensory-evoked activity in the olfactory bulb of LRRK2 knockout mice. Cell 10: 3212. https://doi.org/10.3390/cells10113212
20. Moberly AH, Schreck M, Bhattarai JP, Zweifel LS, Luo W, Ma M (2018) Olfactory inputs modulate respiration-related rhythmic activity in the prefrontal cortex and freezing behavior. Nat Commun 9:1528. https://doi.org/10.1038/s41467-018-03988-1
21. Ruan Y, Zheng X-Y, Zhang H-L, Zhu W, Zhu J (2012) Olfactory dysfunctions in neurodegenerative disorders. J Neurosci Res 90:1693–1700. https://doi.org/10.1002/jnr.23054
22. Salimi M, Tabasi F, Nazari M, Ghazvineh S, Raoufy MR (2022) The olfactory bulb coordinates the ventral hippocampus–medial prefrontal cortex circuit during spatial working memory performance. J Physiol Sci 72:9. https://doi.org/10.1186/s12576-022-00833-5
23. Brondi M, Bruzzone M, Lodovichi C, Dal Maschio M (2022) Optogenetic methods to investigate brain alterations in preclinical models. Cell 11:1848. https://doi.org/10.3390/cells11111848
24. Leopold AV, Shcherbakova DM, Verkhusha VV (2019) Fluorescent biosensors for neurotransmission and neuromodulation: engineering and applications. Front Cell Neurosci 13: 474. https://doi.org/10.3389/fncel.2019.00474
25. Marvin JS, Borghuis BG, Tian L, Cichon J, Harnett MT, Akerboom J, Gordus A, Renninger SL, Chen TW, Bargmann CI et al (2013)

An optimized fluorescent probe for visualizing glutamate neurotransmission. Nat Methods 10:162–170. https://doi.org/10.1038/nmeth.2333

26. Sabatini BL, Tian L (2020) Imaging neurotransmitter and neuromodulator dynamics in vivo with genetically encoded indicators. Neuron 108:17–32. https://doi.org/10.1016/j.neuron.2020.09.036

Chapter 12

Target-Captured mRNA from Murine Olfactory Bulb

Kevin W. Zhu and Hiroaki Matsunami

Abstract

The external world is perceived via sensory receptors arranged in highly organized systems according to functional strategies, which in turn reflect features of critical importance to both the sense and the animal. Thus describing the receptor organization and functional strategies of olfaction, the sense of smell, is crucial for a concrete understanding of the fundamental principles of the system's architecture. Sensory processing in olfactory systems is organized across olfactory bulb (OB) glomeruli, wherein axons of peripheral sensory neurons expressing the same olfactory receptor (OR) co-terminate to transmit receptor-specific activity to mitral/tufted cells, projection neurons in the olfactory bulb. Understanding how receptors map to glomeruli is therefore critical to understanding olfaction.

Here we describe a method to enrich low-abundant OR mRNAs from the mouse OB for spatial transcriptomics to generate high-throughput mapping of receptors to glomeruli [2]. Our method combines sequential sectioning along the anteroposterior, dorsoventral, and mediolateral axes with target capture enrichment sequencing to overcome low-abundance target expression. This strategy spatially mapped 86% of olfactory receptors across the olfactory bulb and uncovered a relationship between olfactory receptor sequence and glomerular position.

Key words Olfactory bulb, Gene expression analysis, Olfactory receptor, RNA sequencing

1 Introduction

The perception of an odor begins when volatile chemical molecules enter the nasal mucosa and bind to olfactory receptors (ORs) on the dendritic cilia of olfactory sensory neurons (OSNs). Once bound, the chemical ligand stabilizes the active conformation of the receptor, resulting in a signaling cascade that triggers OSN depolarization. OSNs expressing the same OR project to the olfactory bulb (OB) where they form discrete, homotypic structures called glomeruli [1, 2]. These glomeruli are innervated by secondary OB neurons, such as mitral cells, which relay information to the olfactory cortex where signals are interpreted and translated into behaviors.

Bradley J. Goldstein and Hiroaki Matsunami (eds.), *The Olfactory System*, Methods in Molecular Biology, vol. 2710, https://doi.org/10.1007/978-1-0716-3425-7_12,

Olfactory receptors are members of the seven transmembrane G protein-coupled receptor (GPCR) superfamily. As members of the Class A rhodopsin-like subfamily, ORs make up the largest gene family in most vertebrates, with total repertoires numbering approximately 1100 in mice. ORs are typically single-exon genes approximately 1000 nucleotides long and located in clusters across 18 chromosomes. in mice the mammalian OR repertoire is divided into the Class I (so called fish-like) ORs (~10% of repertoire in mice) and Class II ORs (~90% of repertoire in mice) based on their evolutionary origins [3, 4].

The olfactory epithelium is stratified thanks to the existence of continuous, overlapping zones of OR expression along the dorsoventral axis of the OE (Fig. 1a). RNA in situ hybridization (ISH) experiments initially suggested the mouse OE is divided into four overlapping zones of OR expression, with zone 1 being the most dorsal and zone 4 the most ventral [5, 6, 7]. More recent studies applying spatial transcriptomic and multiplex RNA ISH have proposed the division of the OE into larger number of zones [8, 9, 10].

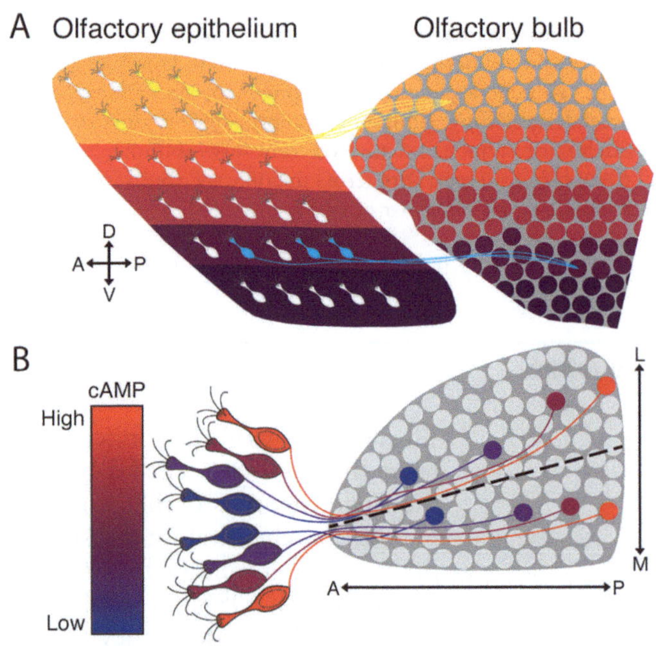

Fig. 1 Axon targeting of olfactory sensory neurons. (**a**) Zonal projection along the dorsoventral axis is dependent upon OSN location in the OE, with OSNs expressing dorsal zone ORs projecting to dorsal OB glomeruli and ventral zone ORs projecting to ventral OB glomeruli. (**b**) Projection of OSNs along the anteroposterior axis depends on OR-specific levels of cAMP which drives expression of axon guidance molecules. OSNs with higher levels of cAMP project to more posterior glomeruli and OSNs with lower levels project to more anterior positions. Projections of OSNs to paired glomeruli located across a line of mirror symmetry are depicted

In situ hybridization experiments probed for specific ORs to determine the organization of olfactory information and revealed that specific OR transcripts were concentrated within only a handful of glomeruli as opposed to distributed throughout all glomeruli [7, 11, 12]. Furthermore, the projection sites for these ORs were consistent in position between individuals. It was also noted that the quantity of OR transcript signal within the OB was extremely low compared to that of OSN somas within the OE, indicating that OR transcripts are in low abundance at the axon terminal. Broad-scale mapping of gene families has found that Class I ORs project to the dorsal, anterior surface of the OB, while Class II ORs project throughout the remaining regions of the OB [13]. Another class of chemosensory receptors, the trace amine-associated receptors (TAARs), has been mapped to a dorsal, central domain. The projection of OSN axons to the OB is an incredible process in which a combination of OR-dependent and OR-independent mechanisms produces a stereotyped spatial organization of OR-specific glomeruli between individuals. Together these studies established the convergence of homotypic OSN axons to stereotyped glomeruli whose positional variability ranges from 75 to 270 μm depending on OR identity [11, 14]. Because each glomerulus represents a single OR and a single odorant can bind multiple ORs, odor signals detected in the OE are transformed into a map of glomerular activity on the OB [15, 16, 17, 18, 19].

A more efficient approach for mapping OR axon projections to OB glomeruli would serve to generate a more comprehensive and informative map that would serve as a foundation for further functional studies of odor coding and processing. To enrich sampling for OR transcripts, we designed a target capture array against chemosensory receptor gene families primarily targeting ORs and TAARs [20] (Fig. 2).

Using the method described below, we demonstrate that target capture enrichment on sequential samples from the OB enables detection of low-abundance OR and TAAR mRNA in the axon termini of OSNs. Using this approach, we map 86% of the 1118 ORs and TAARs along the anteroposterior, mediolateral, and dorsoventral axes and combine these data to generate a three-dimensional model of glomerular positions.

2 Materials

2.1 Reagents

1. Low melting point (LMP) agar (American Bioanalytical, AB00981).
2. Hanks' Balanced Salt Solution (HBSS), no calcium, no magnesium, no phenol red (Gibco, 14175-095).
3. Loctite® 404 glue.

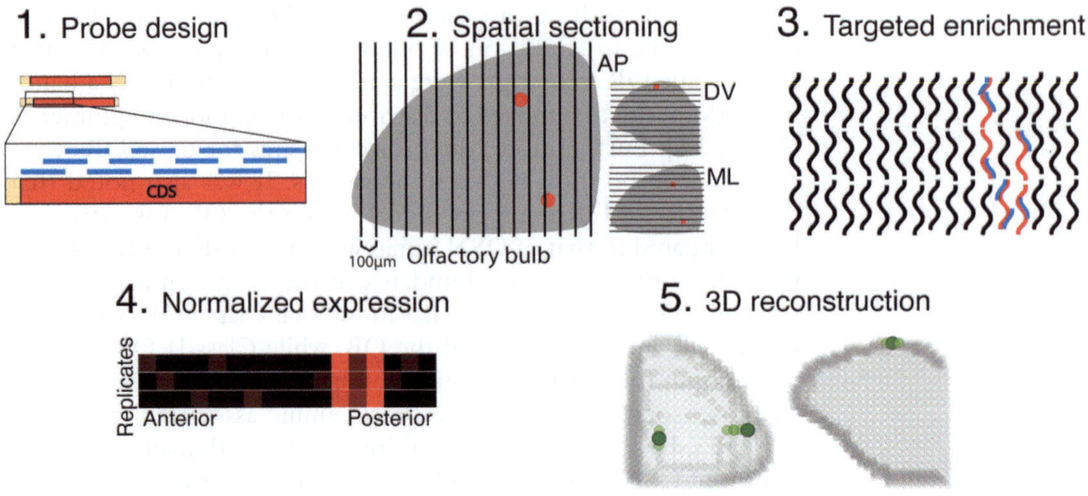

Fig. 2 Method overview for targeted enrichment of OR and TAAR transcripts from OB sections. RNA is extracted from OB sections and used for cDNA synthesis and library preparation. Biotinylated capture probes are designed against coding sequences of interest, enabling enrichment of target genes following streptavidin binding and washing steps. RNA-seq of enriched libraries allows for high-throughput positional analyses when combined with systematic tissue sectioning in both individual dimensions and in 3D after reconstruction

4. Phosphate-buffered saline (PBS) pH 7.4.
5. Bucket of ice.
6. RNeasy Micro Kit (QIAGEN, 74004).
7. Qubit™ RNA High Sensitivity (HS) Assay Kit (Thermo Fisher, Q32852).
8. 200 Proof ethanol.
9. UltraPure™ DNase/RNase-Free Distilled Water (Thermo Fisher, 10977015).
10. SMART-Seq® v4 Ultra Low Input RNA Kit (TaKaRa, 634894).
11. AMPure XP beads (Beckman Coulter, A63881).
12. Qubit™ dsDNA High-Sensitivity (HS) Assay Kit (Thermo Fisher, Q32851).
13. 1 M Tris–HCl pH 8.0.
14. KAPA HyperPlus Library Kit (Roche, KK8514, 07962428001).
15. SeqCap Adapter Kit A (Roche, 07141530001).
16. SeqCap Adapter Kit B (Roche, 07141548001).
17. SeqCap EZ HE-Oligo Kit A (Roche, 06777287001).
18. SeqCap EZ HE-Oligo Kit B (Roche, 06777317001).
19. SeqCap Hybridization and Wash Kit (Roche, 05634261001).
20. SeqCap Accessory Kit v2 (Roche, 07145594001).

21. SeqCap RNA Choice Enrichment Kit (12 reactions) (Roche, 07277300001).
22. QIAquick PCR Purification Kit (QIAGEN, 28104).

2.2 Equipment

1. Water bath.
2. Zeiss Stemi 305 dissection microscope.
3. Dumont #5 forceps (Fine Science Tools, 11252-20).
4. Dissection scissors (McKesson, 421375).
5. Spring scissors (Fine Science Tools, 91500-09).
6. Standard 100 mm x 15 mm petri dishes.
7. Rectangular R30 embedding mold (Peel-A-Way, 18646B-1).
8. Transfer pipettes (Thermo Fisher, 212-20S).
9. Thermometer probe (Thermo Fisher, TS-18915).
10. Leica VT1000S vibratome.
11. Double-edge feather razor blades.
12. Clean single-edge standard razor blades.
13. 1.5 mL tubes (Eppendorf, 022431021).
14. Standard microwave.
15. Eppendorf centrifuge 5424 (Thermo Fisher, 05-400-005).
16. Vortex mixer.
17. Bio-Gen PRO200 homogenizer with 5 flat tip generator probe (PRO Scientific, 01-01200).
18. Qubit™ 2.0 fluorometer (Thermo Fisher, Q32866).
19. Qubit™ Assay Tubes (Thermo Fisher, Q32856).
20. 15 mL conical tubes.
21. 50 mL conical tubes.
22. Kimwipes (Thermo Fisher, 06-666).
23. 1000 μL filtered pipette tips.
24. 200 μL filtered pipette tips.
25. 20 μL filtered pipette tips.
26. 10 μL filtered pipette tips.
27. 8-Strip 0.2 mL PCR tubes.
28. Fisherbrand™ Mini-Centrifuge for 0.2 mL tubes (Fisher Scientific, 12006901).
29. 0.2 mL PCR tube magnetic rack (Alpaqua, A001322).
30. 1.5 mL tube magnetic rack (NEB, S1509S).
31. PCR thermocycler.
32. Dry bath/block heater for 1.5 mL tubes.

33. 18-gauge needle.
34. Savant SC110A-115 SpeedVac Plus Concentrator.

2.3 Solutions

1. 3% LMP Agar in HBSS: Dissection of one olfactory bulb requires 20 mL of solution; add 0.6 g LMP Agar to 20 mL HBSS.
2. 70% ethanol: Combine 14 mL 200 proof ethanol with 6 mL UltraPure™ water to make 20 mL solution. For each sample, 700 μL is required in the OB sectioning and RNA extraction protocols. A 70% ethanol solution is also used for sterilization purposes during olfactory bulb dissection.
3. 80% ethanol: Combine 16 mL 200 proof ethanol with 4 mL UltraPure™ water to make 20 mL. Make fresh for each protocol that requires this solution. RNA extraction requires 500 μL per sample; cDNA synthesis requires 400 μL per sample; sequencing library construction requires 800 μL per sample; target enrichment requires 400 μL per pool.
4. Buffer RLT: Before use, add 960 μL β-mercaptoethanol to 9.6 mL of Buffer RLT from the RNeasy Micro Kit.
5. Tris–HCl buffer: Dilute 10 μL of 1 M Tris–HCl pH 8.0 in 990 μL sterile, UltraPure™ water to create a 10 mM Tris–HCl solution.
6. SeqCap Index Adapter Stock: Resuspend the SeqCap Index Adapter in 50 μL UltraPure™ water.

3 Methods

3.1 Olfactory Bulb Sectioning

The goal of sectioning murine olfactory bulbs (OBs) is to conserve spatial information and mRNA integrity for future RNA sequencing applications.

3.1.1 Vibratome Setup and Experimental Preparation

1. Cut feather razor blade in half, lengthwise, and remove non-blade flanks that remain on either side of the blade.
2. Secure modified feather razor blade half into the Fresh Tissue Blade Clamp of the vibratome using an appropriate screwdriver to complete the Blade Assembly.
3. Locate the Fresh Tissue Tray for the vibratome.
4. Turn on the vibratome, set section thickness to 100 μm, set frequency to 8, and set speed to 5–50.
5. Warm the water bath to 42 °C.
6. Place HBSS on ice.
7. Label one 1.5 mL tube for each section from each mouse that will be dissected.

8. Bring labeled 1.5 mL tubes, individual embedding molds, thermometer probe, petri dishes, 70% ethanol solution, and PBS near vibratome.
9. Warm 3% LMP agar in HBSS in the microwave until agar is melted and place into 42 °C water bath.

3.1.2 Subjects

Male and female C57BL6 mice at the age of 21 days postnatal are utilized for dissection and sectioning of murine olfactory bulbs.

3.1.3 Olfactory Bulb Dissection and Embedding

1. Humanely euthanize mice following the approved Institutional Animal Care and Use Committee (IACUC) protocol for your experiment.
2. Spray mouse with 70% ethanol and wipe clean with a Kimwipe.
3. Using dissection scissors, decapitate the mouse by cutting from the back of the jaw to the back of the skull.
4. Deglove the upper skull.
5. Remove the anterior portion of the skull by making a coronal cut behind the front teeth.
6. Under the dissection scope, carefully cut down the midline of the dorsal skull, from posterior to anterior, with spring scissors.
7. Next, cut along the ventral perimeter of the skull, and remove skull cover to expose the brain and olfactory bulb (OB).
8. Using spring scissors, sever the olfactory nerve as closely as possible to the OB.
9. Disconnect the brain from the base of the skull, transfer the brain to a petri dish filled with PBS, and place dish under dissection scope.
10. Carefully remove traces of the olfactory nerve from the anterior tip of both OBs.
11. Use dissection scissors to sever one of the OBs, and transfer the detached OB to a 1.5 mL tube and freeze at −80 °C.
12. Transfer the OB which is still connected to the brain into an embedding mold.
13. Remove the LMP agar from the water bath, pour LMP agar into the cube to completely cover the OB and brain.
14. Stir the agar with a thermometer probe to fully embed the OB and brain, and orient the OB so that the OB is lengthwise within the rectangular embedding mold.
15. Place the embedding cube with the embedded OB on ice and place next to the vibratome.

3.1.4 Olfactory Bulb Sectioning

1. Cut along the vertices of the embedding mold (from top to bottom) with a clean razor blade so that the plastic mold can be peeled away. Remove the embedded OB + brain agar cube from the opened mold.
2. With a clean razor blade, cut the cube with embedded OB + brain into a pyramid, such that the apex of the pyramid will be where sectioning begins, and the bottom will be where sectioning ends. Directions for anterior-posterior sectioning are below.
   (a) First, form a wide base by cutting from the top down through the back half of the brain; the posterior end of the front half of the brain will serve as the base of the pyramid.
   (b) Then, form a triangular shape by trimming excess agar from the tip of the OB diagonally to a bottom corner of the agar cube. It is desirable to have the widest base of the pyramid as is possible.
3. Place one to two drops of Loctite 404 glue onto the Fresh Tissue Tray so that you may adhere the base of the agar pyramid with the OB to the Tray.
4. Place the base of the OB agar pyramid onto the drops of Loctite glue (e.g., OB should be pointed up for anterior-posterior sectioning), and allow the glue to dry for approximately 1 min.
5. Place the Fresh Tissue Tray with the adhered OB on the vibratome stand and secure the Tray with the locking lever.
6. Add cold HBSS to the Tray until the embedded OB is completely submerged.
7. Turn the vibratome on and ensure the cut size, frequency, and speed settings are correct.
8. Press the "Up" button to lower the Tray and attach the Blade Assembly to the vibratome using the black pin screw.
9. Press the "Up" button to raise the Tray until the Blade Assembly is as close as possible to the apex of the embedded OB agar pyramid.
10. Use the "Forward" button to move the blade to the desired start position.
11. Press the double-headed arrow button to set the start position.
12. Use the "Forward" button to move the blade to the desired stop position.
13. Press the double-headed arrow button to set the stop position.
14. Set the "Single/Cont" button to "Cont" for continuous, repeated sectioning.

15. Press the "Start" button to begin sectioning.
16. Once sectioning begins, remove OB tissue sections with dissection tweezers from the vibratome, and place them into the appropriately labeled 1.5 mL tubes. (Press "Pause" to stop the blade if more time is needed to isolate tissue sections.)

    Note: A transfer pipette can be used to remove a tissue section from the vibratome if retrieving with tweezers in not possible.
17. After sectioning is complete, turn off vibratome, unscrew Blade Assembly, discard used blades, and clean instrument.
18. Briefly centrifuge OB sections in 1.5 mL tubes at 3000 rpm for 2 s in an Eppendorf 5424 centrifuge.
19. Freeze samples at −80 °C until ready for RNA extraction.

    Note: Ensure that the age and sex of the mouse as well as which side of the OB was sectioned and which side is collected whole is recorded.

3.2 RNA Extraction

The goal of this protocol is to extract total RNA from sections of murine olfactory bulb (OB) tissue sections.

3.2.1 Tissue Homogenization

1. Label one 1.5 mL tube for each sample using only the tissue section number, and fill each tube with 350 μL 70% ethanol.
2. Setup and label RNeasy MinElute spin columns from the RNeasy Micro Kit for each tissue sample.
3. Fill three 50 mL conical tubes with sterile, deionized water, and prepare an ice bucket that can hold all sample tubes.
4. Thaw one tube of DNase I from the RNeasy Micro Kit.
5. Add 400 μL RLT buffer to an OB tissue section that was previously frozen at −80 °C.
6. Place homogenizer probe in sample, and gradually increase homogenizer speed to the maximum setting, and hold for 4 s before gradually decreasing speed to a stop.
7. Remove sample from homogenizer, and immediately place on ice.

   Note: Visually examine sample tube after homogenization to ensure that tissue sample has been homogenized. Solution should appear cloudy with opacity dependent on size of section.
8. To clean homogenizer between samples, run the homogenizer at maximum speed in each of the three conicals of deionized water maintaining order conical tube order (conical tube for first wash, second wash, and third wash). Following the three washes, wipe homogenizer probe with a Kimwipe, turn

homogenizer on to max speed for 5 s, turn off, then wipe again with Kimwipe.

Note: It is recommended to change DI water and/or the wash conicals as frequently as possible.

9. Homogenize all samples, cleaning the homogenizer between each, and then clean the homogenizer one final time to finish.

3.2.2 RNA Extraction

1. Briefly spin homogenized tissue samples in 1.5 mL tubes at maximum speed.

   Note: Steps 1–5 can be performed in a 4 °C cold room for optimal processing of a large number of samples.
2. Transfer 350 μL of supernatant to the correspondingly labeled 1.5 mL tube with 350 μL 70% ethanol that was previously prepared.
3. Mix sample to homogeneity by pipetting up and down several times.
4. Transfer entire sample to appropriately labeled RNeasy column.
5. Centrifuge column in a collection tube for 30 s at 12,000 rpm and discard flow-through.
6. Prepare a DNase solution by combining 10 μL DNase I and 70 μL Buffer RDD for each sample; invert DNase solution to mix.
7. Add 80 μL DNase solution to the RNeasy column and incubate at room temperature for 15 min.
8. Prepare and label two new RNeasy collection tubes for each sample with subject and section number as well as one final, labeled 1.5 mL tube.
9. Add 350 μL Buffer RW1 to the RNeasy column, centrifuge at 12,000 rpm for 30 s, and discard flow-through.
10. Add 500 μL Buffer RPE to the RNeasy column, centrifuge at 12,000 rpm for 30 s, and discard flow-through.
11. Add 500 μL fresh 80% ethanol to the RNeasy column, centrifuge at 12,000 rpm for 2 min, and discard both the flow-through and collection tube.
12. Place column into a new collection tube, and centrifuge at maximum speed for 5 min with the column lid open.
13. Discard flow-through and collection tube, and place column into the final, labeled 1.5 mL tube.
14. Add 14 μL UltraPure™ water to the center of the column and incubate at room temperature for 5 min.
15. Centrifuge column in final 1.5 mL tube at maximum speed for 2 min. Discard RNeasy column.

3.2.3 RNA Quantification

1. Label one Qubit™ Assay tube for each sample and an additional tubes for each assay standard.
2. In a 15 mL conical tube, make the Qubit™ RNA HS MasterMix by combining 5.2 mL Qubit™ RNA HS Buffer and 26 μL Qubit™ RNA HS Reagent; vortex to mix.
3. Add 190 μL MasterMix to the two standard tubes and 199 μL MasterMix to each sample tube.
4. Add 10 μL of each Qubit™ RNA HS Standard to the appropriately labeled standard tube.
5. Add 1 μL RNA sample to the appropriately labeled sample tube.
6. Vortex each tube for 2–3 s and incubate tubes at room temperature for 2 min.
7. Use the Qubit™ fluorometer to first quantify the new standard tubes and then quantify RNA in all sample tubes, recording RNA concentrations for all tubes.
8. Store samples at −80 °C.

3.3 cDNA Synthesis

This protocol is written for the preparation of 24 cDNA reactions (23 samples and one control). Controls typically include either a positive control (10 ng RNA) or a negative control (no RNA). This protocol is adapted from the manufacturer's protocol for the SMART-Seq v4 Ultra Low Input RNA Kit for Sequencing (Takara Clontech).

3.3.1 First-Strand cDNA Synthesis

1. Thaw RNase Inhibitor, 3' SMART-Seq CDS Primer II A, SMART-Seq v4 Oligonucleotide, and SMARTScribe Reverse Transcriptase on ice. Thaw 5X Ultra Low First-Strand Buffer and 10X Lysis Buffer at room temperature.
2. Setup a "72 °C incubation" thermocycler program that will hold at 4 °C until ready, then incubate samples at 72 °C for 3 min before returning to a 4 °C hold. Initiate "72 °C incubation" program to pre-chill thermocycler block.
3. In a PCR strip tube add 25.5 μL of 10X Lysis Buffer and 1.35 μL of RNase Inhibitor to make 10X Reaction Buffer. Mix by pipetting up and down gently.

   Note: Lysis Buffer contains a detergent, avoid bubbles when mixing.
4. Briefly spin 10X Reaction Buffer.
5. Thaw RNA samples and dilute RNA in sterile UltraPure™ water to make a 4.75 μL solution containing 10 μg of total RNA in 8-strip PCR tubes.
6. Add 0.5 μL 10X Reaction Buffer to each sample, and then place on ice.

7. Add 1 μL 3' SMART-Seq CDS Primer II A to each sample and mix by gently tapping the tubes before spinning briefly.
8. Place samples into thermocycler and allow program to move on to 72 °C incubation step.
9. Vortex reagents until thoroughly mixed. Mix SMARTScribe Reverse Transcriptase by tapping tube or pipetting up and down.

    Note: The 5X Ultra Low First-Strand Buffer may form precipitates. Ensure any precipitate is fully dissolved by mixing well.
10. To a new PCR tube, prepare a first-strand mastermix by adding 50 μL 5X Ultra Low First-Strand Buffer, 12.5 μL SMART-Seq v4 Oligonucleotide, 6.25 μL RNase Inhibitor, and 25 μL SMARTScribe Reverse Transcriptase. Pipette up and down to mix before spinning briefly. Keep on ice.
11. Once samples have returned to 4 °C, remove samples from thermocycler and immediately place on ice for 2 min.
12. Add 3.75 μL of first-strand mastermix to each sample. Mix by gently pipetting up and down then spin briefly.
13. Setup a "42 °C incubation" thermocycler program that will hold at 4 °C until ready, incubate samples at 42 °C for 90 min, then incubate samples at 70 °C for 10 min before returning to a 4 °C hold. Initiate "42 °C incubation" program to pre-chill thermocycler block.
14. Place samples into thermocycler and allow program to move on to 42 °C incubation step.

    Note: At this stage samples may be stored at 4 °C or − 20 °C; however, it is optimal to proceed to cDNA amplification.

3.3.2 cDNA Amplification

1. Thaw 2X SeqAmp PCR Buffer, PCR Primer II A, and SeqAmp DNA polymerase on ice.
2. Generate a "cDNA amplification" thermocycler program with the following steps:
    (a) Initial denaturation, 95 °C, 1 min.
    (b) Denaturation, 98 °C, 10 s.
    (c) Annealing, 65 °C, 30 s.
    (d) Extension, 68 °C, 3 min.
    (e) Repeat steps b through d an additional ten times, for a total of 11 cycles.
    (f) Final extension, 72 °C, 10 min.
    (g) 4 °C hold.

3. Mix 2X SeqAmp PCR Buffer and PCR Primer II A by vortexing. Mix SeqAmp DNA polymerase by tapping tube or pipetting up and down.
4. To a new 1.5 mL tube, prepare an amplification mastermix by adding 325 μL 2X SeqAmp PCR Buffer, 39 μL Nuclease-Free water, 13 μL PCR Primer II A, and 13 μL SeqAmp DNA polymerase. Pipette up and down to mix before spinning briefly. Keep on ice.
5. Aliquot 15 μL of amplification mastermix to new PCR strip tubes.
6. Add 10 μL of first-strand cDNA product to each tube with amplification mastermix.
7. Place tubes in thermocycler, and initiate "cDNA amplification" program.
8. Run a check gel by adding 5 μL of sample mixed with 2 μL of dye and running at 100 V for 12 min.
9. Amplified cDNAs should appear as smear signals between 0.5 and 3 kb.

   Note: At this stage samples may be stored at 4 °C overnight or −20 °C for longer periods.

3.3.3 cDNA Purification

1. Bring AMPure XP beads to room temperature for 30 min.
2. Add 0.4 μL of 10X Lysis Buffer to each sample.
3. Vortex AMPure XP beads for 30 s.
4. Add 25 μL AMPure XP beads to each sample tube. Pipette up and down slowly ten times to thoroughly mix.
5. Incubate samples for 10 min at room temperature.
6. Place tubes on magnetic rack for 5 min.

   Note: Tubes will remain on the magnetic rack until elution buffer is added.
7. After the 5 min incubation, while tubes are still on magnetic rack, remove and discard supernatant.
8. Add 200 μL fresh 80% ethanol to each sample on magnetic rack, and incubate for 30 s.
9. Remove supernatant, add 200 μL 80% ethanol, and incubate an additional 30 s.
10. Remove supernatant and air-dry samples with caps open for 2 min or until all ethanol has evaporated.
11. Remove tubes from magnetic rack and add 27 μL elution buffer to each sample. Incubate 5 min at room temperature.
12. Return tubes to magnetic rack, and incubate an additional 5 min.

13. While tubes are still on magnetic rack, transfer 50 μL of adapter-ligated library to a new 1.5 mL tube.
14. Prepare samples for quantification using the Qubit™ dsDNA HS Assay Kit following the same steps described in protocol 3.2.3 but with the dsDNA HS reagents.
15. Quantify and record DNA concentrations of samples.
16. Store samples at −20 °C.

3.4 DNA Sequencing Library Construction

The purpose of this protocol is to use a minimal amount of cDNA to create KAPA Libraries for use in full-size, multiplexed (24 samples) sequence capture. Amplification cycles can be adjusted for the size of the sequence capture and the number of samples to be captured.

3.4.1 cDNA Fragmentation

1. Thaw KAPA Frag Buffer and KAPA Frag Enzyme on ice.
2. Thaw input DNA and dilute DNA in 10 mM Tris–HCl Buffer to make a 35 μL solution containing 10 μg of DNA in 8-strip PCR tubes.
3. Setup a "Fragmentation" thermocycler program that will hold at 4 °C until ready, then incubate samples at 37 °C for 10 min, before returning to a 4 °C hold. Initiate "Fragmentation" program to pre-chill thermocycler block.
4. Add 5 μL KAPA Frag Buffer and then 10 μL KAPA Frag Enzyme to each sample. Vortex to mix.
5. Briefly spin samples in mini-centrifuge and then place on ice.
6. Place samples into thermocycler, and allow program to move on to 37 °C incubation step.
7. Once samples have returned to 4 °C, remove samples from thermocycler and immediately place on ice.

3.4.2 End Repair and A-Tailing

1. Thaw End Repair and A-Tailing Buffer to room temperature as well as End Repair and A-Tailing Enzymes on ice.
2. To each sample tube, add 7 μL of End Repair and A-Tailing Buffer and 3 μL of End Repair and A-Tailing Enzyme. Vortex to mix.
3. Briefly spin samples in mini-centrifuge and place on ice.
4. Create a "Repair-Tailing" thermocycler program that will incubate samples at 65 °C for 30 min, and then move to a 4 °C hold with the lid of the thermocycler heated to 85 °C.
5. Place samples into thermocycler and initiate the "Repair-Tailing" program created in the previous step.
6. Once samples have reached 4 °C in the thermocycler, remove samples, and place immediately on ice.

3.4.3 Adapter Ligation

1. Thaw ligation buffer, DNA ligase, and SeqCap Index Adapter. (If necessary, resuspend SeqCap Index Adapter in 50 μL of sterile UltraPure™ water.)
2. To a new PCR tube (one per sample), add 5 μL sterile UltraPure™ water, 30 μL Ligation Bugger, and 10 μL DNA ligase to make the Ligation Premix.
3. Record the barcode adapters used for each library.
4. To each sample, add 0.75 μL SeqCap Index Adapter Stock and 45 μL of the Ligation Premix. Pipette up and down five times to mix.
5. Briefly spin samples in a mini-centrifuge.
6. Generate a "Ligation" thermocycler program to incubate sample at 10 °C for 90 min.
7. Move samples to thermocycler and initiate "Ligation" program.
8. Record use of SeqCap Index Adapter.
9. After incubation is complete, remove samples from thermocycler, and place on ice.

3.4.4 Bead Purification of Adapter-Ligated Library

1. Bring AMPure XP beads to room temperature for 30 min.
2. Thaw Library Amplification Primer Mix and KAPA HiFi Hotstart ReadyMix.
3. Vortex AMPure XP beads for 30 s.
4. Add 88 μL AMPure XP beads to each sample tube. Pipette up and down slowly ten times to thoroughly mix.
5. Incubate samples for 10 min at room temperature.
6. Place tubes on magnetic rack for 5 min.

   Note: Tubes will remain on the magnetic rack until elution buffer is added.
7. After the 5 min incubation, while tubes are still on magnetic rack, remove and discard supernatant.
8. Add 200 μL fresh 80% ethanol to each sample on magnetic rack, and incubate for 30 s.
9. Remove supernatant, add 200 μL 80% ethanol, and incubate an additional 30 s.
10. Remove supernatant and air-dry samples with caps open for 3 min or until all ethanol has evaporated.
11. Remove tubes from magnetic rack and add 55 μL elution buffer to each sample. Incubate 5 min at room temperature.
12. Return tubes to magnetic rack and incubate an additional 5 min.

13. While tubes are still on magnetic rack, transfer 50 μL of adapter-ligated library to a new 1.5 mL tube.
14. Tubes with adapter-ligated library can be stored at −20 °C if not continuing.

3.4.5 Library Amplification

1. Generate an "Amplification" thermocycler program with the following steps:
   (a) Initial denaturation, 98 °C, 45 s.
   (b) Denaturation, 98 °C, 15 s.
   (c) Annealing, 60 °C, 30 s.
   (d) Extension, 72 °C, 30 s.
   (e) Repeat steps b through d an additional five times, for a total of six cycles.
   (f) Final extension, 72 °C, 1 min.
   (g) 4 °C hold.

   Note: The library amplification output is dependent on original input, fragmentation time, and cycles. With this protocol, 6 cycles will produce approximately 80 ng of DNA (enough for 2 captures of 24 samples).
2. To a new PCR tube, add 25 μL KAPA HiFi HotStart ReadyMix.
3. To the same tube, add 5 μL Library Amplification Primer Mix and 20 μL of adapter-ligated library, and pipette up and down five times to mix.
4. Briefly spin tubes in a mini-centrifuge.
5. Place tubes in thermocycler and initiate "Amplification" program.

3.4.6 Bead Purification of Amplified Library

1. Vortex AMPure XP beads for 30 s.
2. Add 50 μL AMPure XP beads to each PCR sample tube. Pipette up and down ten times, slowly.
3. Incubate samples at room temperature for 10 min.
4. Place samples on PCR tube magnetic rack for 5 min.

   Note: Samples will remain on the magnetic rack for the following steps until after samples have been air-dried.
5. Remove and discard supernatant.
6. Wash samples twice with 200 μL fresh 80% ethanol, incubating for samples for 30 s in ethanol for each wash step.
7. Remove and discard supernatant and allow samples to air-dry with caps open for 3 min or until all ethanol has evaporated.
8. Remove samples from magnetic rack.

9. Add 25 μL UltraPure™ water to each tube and incubate at room temperature for 5 min.
10. Prepare samples for quantification using the Qubit™ dsDNA HS Assay Kit following the same steps described in protocol 3.2.3 but with the dsDNA HS reagents.
11. Quantify DNA concentrations of samples.
12. Store samples at −20 °C.

3.5 Enrichment of Target Sequences

The purpose of this protocol is to enrich RNA-seq libraries for transcript cDNAs of interest through hybridization to a biotinylated probe array. This protocol has been adjusted for half-size reactions to increase productivity of the kit. Protocol is adapted from the SeqCap RNA Enrichment System User's Guide v1.0.

3.5.1 Probe Hybridization

1. Thaw KAPA amplified libraries to room temperature.
2. On ice, thaw 100 μM SeqCap HE Universal Oligo and SeqCap Probe Pool as well as the 2X Hybridization Buffer and Hybridization Component A from the SeqCap Hybridization and Wash Kit.
3. Aliquot 4.5 μL of the SeqCap Probe Pool into 0.2 mL PCR tubes. (Remaining aliquots can be stored at −20 °C for future use.)
4. Preheat a dry block heater to 95 °C.
5. Calculate the DNA quantity of each library to add to the pool by dividing 1000 ng by the number of libraries. Then calculate the volume of each library needed for the pool based on previous library DNA quantification.
6. Add the calculated volume of each library to a single 1.5 mL library pool tube.

   Note: If library pool volume is greater than 57 μL, purify using a QIAGEN PCR Purification Kit: Add 5 volumes Buffer PB, splitting if necessary. Pipette mixture up and down 5X to mix. Load 750 μL of the library pool + Buffer PB mixture into MinElute column and centrifuge at maximum speed for 1 min. Discard flow-through into a spare tube (in case of massive DNA loss). Repeat until the full library pool + Buffer PB mixture has been centrifuged through the column. Add 750 μL Buffer PE, and centrifuge at maximum speed for 1 min. Discard flow-through and place column in a new 1.5 mL tube. Add 10 μL Buffer EB to column, let stand at room temperature for 1 min, and centrifuge at maximum speed for 1 min. Save column and use Qubit™ fluorometer with the Qubit™ dsDNA HS Assay Kit to quantify DNA in eluate.

7. Add 5 μL COT Human DNA (1 mg/mL) from the SeqCap Accessory Kit v2 to a new 1.5 mL tube. and add the entire library pool volume to this new tube.
8. Use a needle to poke a hole in a new cap of a different, new 1.5 mL tube; remove cap from tube.
9. Close the 1.5 mL tube with the library pool and COT Human DNA with the severed cap with hole, leaving the primary cap of the tube attached and intact.
10. Place tube with library pool into the SpeedVac and concentrate DNA at +60 °C (high heat) until sample is dry (approximately 30 min).
11. Add 7.5 μL 2X Hybridization Buffer to the library pool tube.
12. Remove severed tube lid with hole, and use attached, intact lid for remainder of protocol.
13. Vortex library pool for 10 s, and centrifuge at maximum speed for 10 s.
14. Incubate library pool on 95 °C dry block heater for 10 min.
15. Centrifuge library pool at maximum speed for 10 s.
16. Transfer library pool to a 0.2 mL tube with a SeqCap Probe Pool aliquot.
17. Vortex probe for 3 s, and centrifuge at maximum speed for 10 s.
18. On a thermocycler, create a "Capture" program that will incubate samples at 47 °C indefinitely.
19. Place sample into thermocycler and initiate "Capture" program.
20. After 16 to 20 hours has elapsed, remove samples from thermocycler, and proceed immediately to Target Transcript Recovery protocol. Do not turn off thermocycler.

    Note: Experimental preparation for the next portion of the protocol should begin approximately 2 hours before the 47 °C incubation of the library pool is complete.

3.5.2 Target Transcript Recovery

1. Preheat a dry block heater to 47 °C.
2. Thaw Capture Beads from the SeqCap Accessory Kit at room temperature for at least 30 min prior to vortexing.
3. In a 1.5 mL tube, dilute 40 μL of 10X Stringent Wash Buffer in 360 μL of UltraPure™ water to create 1X Stringent Wash Buffer.
4. In a 1.5 mL tube, dilute 30 μL of 10X Wash Buffer 1 in 270 μL of UltraPure™ water to create 1X Wash Buffer 1.
5. Dilute 20 μL of 10X Wash Buffer 2 in 180 μL of UltraPure™ water to create 1X Wash Buffer 2.

6. Dilute 20 μL of 10X Wash Buffer 3 in 180 μL of UltraPure™ water to create 1X Wash Buffer 3.
7. Dilute 200 μL of 2.5X Bead Wash Buffer in 300 μL of UltraPure™ water to create 1X Bead Wash Buffer.
8. Place 1X Stringent Wash Buffer and 1X Wash Buffer 1 into 47 °C heat block to incubate for 2 hours before use. (Preparation of DNA library will take at least 45 min before wash buffers will be used.)
9. Vortex Capture Beads for 15 s, transfer 100 μL of beads to a new 1.5 mL tube, and place tube in magnetic rack.
10. Once beads have conglomerated, with tube still on magnetic rack, remove and discard supernatant.
11. Add 200 μL 1X Bead Wash Buffer to tube on magnetic rack.
12. Remove tube from magnetic rack and vortex for 10 s.
13. Return tube to magnetic rack, and once beads have compacted, remove and discard supernatant.
14. Repeat steps 11 through 13 once more to wash beads a second time.
15. Add 100 μL 1X Bead Wash Buffer to beads, remove from magnetic rack, and vortex until resuspended.
16. Transfer bead solution to a 0.2 mL PCR tube, and place tube in magnetic rack. (Do not discard supernatant until ready to bind hybridization samples.)
17. Remove library pool from thermocycler, leaving thermocycler on, and check for excessive evaporation (at least 12.5 μL of sample should remain).
18. Discard supernatant from PCR tube with beads on the magnetic rack, and transfer entire library pool volume to tube with beads.
19. Remove tube from magnetic rack, pipette sample up and down 10X to mix, and place tube in 47 °C thermocycler.
20. For 45 min, vortex library pool tube for 3 s every 15 min (3 rounds of vortexing).
21. Add 100 μL 1X Wash Buffer 1 to library pool tube, vortex for 10 s, and transfer entire volume to a new 1.5 mL tube.
22. Place 1.5 mL tube with sample on magnetic rack.
23. Once beads have compacted and solution is clear, remove supernatant while tube is still on magnetic rack.
24. Remove tube from magnetic rack, add 200 μL 1X Stringent Wash Buffer, and pipette up and down 10X to mix.
25. Return sample to 47 °C thermocycler and incubate for 5 min.

26. Place sample on magnetic rack and remove and discard supernatant once beads compact and solution becomes clear.
27. Repeat steps 24 through 26 once more for a second wash.
28. Add 200 μL room temperature 1X Wash Buffer 1 to tube, vortex for 2 min.
29. Tap tube to dislodge any solution from the lid, return the tube to the magnetic rack, and discard supernatant once beads compact.
30. Add 200 μL room temperature 1X Wash Buffer 2, vortex 1 min.
31. Tap tube to dislodge any solution from the lid, return the tube to the magnetic rack, and discard supernatant once beads compact.
32. Add 200 μL room temperature 1X Wash Buffer 3, vortex 30 s.
33. Tap tube to dislodge any solution from the lid, return the tube to the magnetic rack, and discard supernatant once beads compact.
34. Remove tube from magnetic rack, and add 50 μL UltraPure™ water to the captured library, leaving beads with the eluate.
35. Captured library sample can be stored at −20 °C.

3.5.3 Ligation-Mediated (LM) PCR Amplification

1. On ice, thaw captured library sample, KAPA HiFi HotStart ReadyMix (2X), and 5 μM Pre LM-PCR Oligos 1 and 2.
2. Make a master mix with 55 μL ReadyMix and 5.5 μL of each LM-PCR oligo, pipette up and down 10X to mix, and add 30 μL master mix each to two 0.2 mL PCR tubes.
3. Pulse vortex the thawed captured library for 15 s.
4. Add 20 μL of the captured library (including beads) to each of the PCR tubes.
5. Modify the "Amplification" thermocycler program previously generated (Subheading 3.4.5) to repeat steps b through d eight times, for a total of nine cycles.
6. Place PCR tubes in thermocycler, and run the modified "Amplification" program.
7. After thermocycler program is complete, proceed to LM-PCR Purification, or reactions can be stored at 4 °C for up to 72 h.

3.5.4 LM-PCR Purification

1. Thaw the AMPure XP beads to room temperature.
2. Vortex AMPure XP beads for 30 s.
3. Combine both LM-PCR reaction volumes into a single 1.5 mL tube.

4. Add 180 μL to the 1.5 mL tube and pulse vortex sample five times.
5. Incubate the sample at room temperature for 15 min.
6. Place 1.5 mL tube on magnetic rack and, once beads have compacted and solution is clear, remove and discard supernatant.

   Note: Leave sample on magnetic rack for the following steps until after sample has air-dried.
7. Add 200 μL fresh 80% ethanol to sample, and incubate for 30 s at room temperature.
8. Remove and discard supernatant.
9. Repeat steps 6 and 7 for a second 80% ethanol wash.
10. Allow the beads to air-dry for 3 min or until all ethanol has evaporated.
11. Remove tube from magnetic rack, and add 52 μL UltraPure™ water.
12. Pipette mixture up and down ten times to resuspend beads, and incubate at room temperature for 2 min.
13. Place tube in magnetic rack.
14. Once beads have compacted and solution has cleared, transfer 50 μL of supernatant to a new 1.5 mL tube. This is the final target-enriched pool.
15. Use a Qubit™ fluorometer and the Qubit™ dsDNA HS Assay Kit to quantify the DNA in the pool. If DNA quantity is inadequate, add an additional 10 μL UltraPure™ water to the pool, and repeat the LM-PCR Amplification and LM-PCR Purification protocols a second time.

References

1. Wang IH, Murray E, Andrews G, Jiang HC, Park SJ, Donnard E, Durán-Laforet V, Bear DM, Faust TE, Garber M, Baer CE, Schafer DP, Weng Z, Chen F, Macosko EZ, Greer PL (2022) Spatial transcriptomic reconstruction of the mouse olfactory glomerular map suggests principles of odor processing. Nat Neurosci 25(4):484–492
2. Zhu KW, Burton SD, Silverman JD, de March CA, Wachowiak M, Matsunami H (2022) Decoding the olfactory map through targeted transcriptomics links murine olfactory receptors to glomeruli. Nat Commun 13:5137
3. Zhang X, Rodriguez I, Mombaerts P, Firestein S (2004) Odorant and vomeronasal receptor genes in two mouse genome assemblies. Genomics 83(5):802–811
4. Niimura Y (2009) Evolutionary dynamics of olfactory receptor genes in chordates: interaction between environments and genomic contents. Hum Genomics 4:107
5. Ressler KJ, Sullivan SL, Buck LB (1993) A zonal organization of odorant receptor gene expression in the olfactory epithelium. Cell 73:597–609
6. Vassar R, Ngai J, Axel R (1993) Spatial segregation of odorant receptor expression in the mammalian olfactory epithelium. Cell 74: 308–318
7. Miyamachi K, Serizawa S, Kimura HM, Sakano H (2005) Continue and overlapping

expression domains of odorant receptor genes in the olfactory epithelium determine the dorsal/ventral positioning of glomeruli in the olfactory bulb. J Neurosci 24:3586–3592

8. Tan L, Xie XS (2018) A near-complete spatial map of olfactory receptors in the mouse main olfactory epithelium. Chem Senses 43(6): 427–432
9. Zapiec B, Mombaerts P (2020) The zonal organization of odorant receptor gene choice in the main olfactory epithelium of the mouse. Cell Rep 30:4220–4234
10. Ruiz Tejada Segura ML, Abou Moussa E, Garabello E, Nakahara TS, Makhlouf M, Mathew LS, Wang L, Valle F, Huang SSY, Mainland JD, Caselle M, Osella M, Lorenz S, Reisert J, Logan DW, Malnic B, Scialdone A, Saraiva LR (2022) A 3D transcriptomics atlas of the mouse nose sheds light on the anatomical logic of smell. Cell Rep 38(12):110547
11. Ressler KJ, Sullivan SL, Buck LB (1994) Information coding in the olfactory system: evidence for a stereotyped and highly organized epitope map in the olfactory bulb. Cell 79: 1245–1255
12. Vassar R, Chao SK, Sitcheran R, Nuñez JM, Vosshall LB, Axel R (1994) Topographic organization of sensory projections to the olfactory bulb. Cell 79(6):981–991
13. Bozza T, Vassalli A, Fuss S, Zhang JJ, Weiland B, Pacifico R, Feinstein P, Mombaerts P (2009) Mapping of class I and class II odorant receptors to glomerular domains by two distinct types of olfactory sensory neurons in the mouse. Neuron 61:220–233
14. Zapiec B, Mombaerts P (2015) Multiplex assessment of the positions of odorant receptor-specific glomeruli in the mouse olfactory bulb by serial two-photon tomography. Proc Natl Acad Sci U S A 112(43):5873–5882
15. Friedrich RW, Korsching SI (1997) Combinatorial and chemotopic odorant coding in the zebrafish olfactory bulb visualized by optical imaging. Neuron 18(5):737–752
16. Rubin BD, Katz LC (1999) Optical imaging of odorant representations in the mammalian olfactory bulb. Neuron 23(3):499–511
17. Wachowiak M, Cohen LB (2001) Representation of odorants by receptor neuron input to the mouse olfactory bulb. Neuron 32(4): 723–735
18. Bozza T, McGann JP, Mombaerts P, Wachowiak M (2004) In vivo imaging of neuronal activity by targeted expression of a genetically encoded probe in the mouse. Neuron 42(1): 9–21
19. Oka T, Katayama K, Hansman GS, Kageyama T, Ogawa S, Wu FT, White PA, Takeda N (2006) Detection of human sapovirus by real-time reverse transcription-polymerase chain reaction. J Med Virol 78: 1347–1353
20. Mercer TR, Clark MB, Crawford J, Brunck ME, Gerhardt DJ, Taft RJ, Nielsen LK, Dinger ME, Mattick JS (2014) Targeted sequencing for gene discovery and quantification using RNA CaptureSeq. Nat Protoc 9(5):989–1009

Chapter 13

Identification and Localization of Cell Types in the Mouse Olfactory Bulb Using Slide-SeqV2

Ai Fang, Kaitlyn Petentler, Andrew Price, Seth Malloy, Michael Peterson, Lucinda Maddera, Jonathon Russell, McKenzie Treese, Hua Li, Yongfu Wang, Sean McKinney, Anoja Perera, and C. Ron Yu

Abstract

Spatial transcriptomics maps RNA molecules to the location in a tissue where they are expressed. Here we document the use of Slide-SeqV2 to visualize gene expression in the mouse olfactory bulb (OB). This approach relies on spatially identified beads to locate and quantify individual transcripts. The expression profiles associated with the beads are used to identify and localize individual cell types in an unbiased manner. We demonstrate the various cell types and subtypes with distinct spatial locations in the olfactory bulb that are identified using Slide-SeqV2.

Key words Slide-SeqV2, Olfactory bulb, Neural development, GABAergic interneurons, Mitral and tufted cells, Spatial transcriptome, Mouse

1 Introduction

Advances in next-generation sequencing (NGS) technologies have revolutionized how cells are identified and characterized. Bulk and single-cell transcriptome profiling has enabled studies of gene expression in the olfactory tissues of vertebrate species to elucidate developmental changes and identify various cell types [1–9]. In single cell or single nucleus transcriptomics, RNA molecules from dissociated cells or nuclei are tagged, amplified, and sequenced to determine expression profiles of individual cells [10, 11]. Cells sharing similar gene expression profiles can be clustered statistically and identified as specific types based on known markers [12]. The dissociation process, however, has led to the loss of spatial information of

The original version of this chapter was revised. The correction to this chapter is available at https://doi.org/10.1007/978-1-0716-3425-7_17

Bradley J. Goldstein and Hiroaki Matsunami (eds.), *The Olfactory System*, Methods in Molecular Biology, vol. 2710, https://doi.org/10.1007/978-1-0716-3425-7_13,

cells. Moreover, rare cells may not be efficiently captured from the dissociated cell population, which can result in the underrepresentation, or the complete absence, of these cells in the final analysis.

To overcome these limitations, multiple technology platforms have been developed to preserve information of cells in the tissue context. For example, several single-cell, high-plex imaging platforms have been used to identify cell clusters and reveal spatial relationships between cells [13–21]. However, these platforms are limited in the number of genes to be quantified, which must be manually curated. Spatial transcriptomics, on the other hand, relies on localized RNA capturing followed by sequencing to provides a comprehensive survey of all transcripts in the cells [22–24]. In Slide-SeqV2, for example, beads coated with oligonucleotides are used to capture and process mRNA by tethering mRNA molecules onto the beads for reverse transcription, followed by amplification and sequencing. Once sequenced, the spatial barcodes on the oligo allow post hoc assignment of the sequenced molecules to individual beads, such that the mRNA species can be quantified and mapped to specific locations. This method not only preserves the spatial information but also provides an unbiased analysis of transcriptomes.

In the developing olfactory system, olfactory sensory axons project into the olfactory bulb (OB) to innervate their target glomeruli [25–27]. Sensory axons undergo a change in the level of plasticity during the first postnatal week, defined as the critical period [3, 28–30]. Coincidentally, the OB also undergoes a dramatic change during the first postnatal week. For example, the mitral tufted cells prune their primary dendrites [28, 31–33]. Different types of GABAergic interneurons mature during this period [34, 35]. Whereas multiple types of interneuron types have been described, the molecular composition that defines these cells remain unknown. Therefore, we use Slide-SeqV2 to perform unbiased cell clustering and map the cell clusters onto the olfactory bulb [36, 37].We have used this approach to identify a new class of neurons in the olfactory epithelium [38]. Here we describe the procedure to perform Slide-SeqV2 on a P7 OB section and the analysis that follows.

2 Materials

1. Anesthetic Reagent: dissolve 2 g urethane (Sigma, U2500) in 10 mL 1x PBS (pH = 7.4, Gibco, 10010023). Store at room temperature.

   (*Reagents 2–7 must be RNase free.*)

2. Hank's Balanced Salt Solution (HBSS, 1x), without calcium, magnesium, or phenol red (VWR Life Science, 02-0121-0500).
3. O.C.T. (Sakura, 4583), embedding medium for frozen tissue specimens.

4. Pre-sequenced Slide-Seq Pucks. Pucks used in this study were generated and sequenced at the Broad Institute (Cambridge, MA) as described in the Methods and Supplementary Information section of the Slide-SeqV2 publication [37]. The pucks were received on small glass coverslips in 1.7 mL LoBind tubes. Pucks need to be stored at 4 °C after receiving.
5. SSC Buffer (20X concentrate): dissolve 175.3 g NaCl and 88.2 g sodium citrate•2H2O in 800 mL DEPC-treated water. Use citric acid to adjust the pH to 5. Adjust the volume to 1 L with DEPC-treated water. Autoclave and store at room temperature.
6. Hybridization Buffer: add 2unit/μL RNase inhibitor (Lucigen NxGen, F83923–1) into 6x SSC buffer. 200 μL per puck. Prepare before use.
7. Reverse Transcription (RT) Solution: 115 μL DEPC-treated water, 40 μL 5X Maxima RT buffer (Thermo Fisher, EP0753), 20 μL 10 mM dNTPs (NEB, N0477L), 5 μL RNase inhibitor (Lucigen NxGen, F83923–1), 10 μL 50 μM Template Switch Oligo (custom from IDT [see sequence below on 20]), 10 μL Maxima H-RTase (Thermo Fisher, EP0753). 200 μL per puck. Prepare before use.

   (*The following reagents need to be DNase free.*)
8. 2X Tissue Digestion Buffer: add 100 mM Tris–HCl pH 8.0, 200 mM NaCl, 2% SDS, 5 mM EDTA, and 32 unit/μL proteinase K (NEB, P8107S) in autoclaved ddH_2O. Prepare before use.
9. Wash Buffer: add 10 mM Tris–HCl pH 8.0, 1 mM EDTA, and 0.01% Tween-20 in autoclaved ddH_2O. Prepare before use.
10. 10 mM Tris–HCl (pH 8.0): for 10 mM Tris–HCl, dilute 1 M solution (Thermo Fisher, 15568025) 1:100 with DEPC water. Prepare before use. This solution is used at Subheading 3.3, **step 6**, for library preparation.
11. Exonuclease I Solution: Add 20 μL ExoI buffer and 10 μL ExoI (NEB, M0568L) to 170 μL autoclaved ddH_2O. Prepare before use.
12. 0.1 N NaOH (Fisher Scientific, S25549). Store at room temperature.
13. Tris–EDTA Buffer (TE buffer; Thermo Fisher, AM9849).
14. Second Strand Mix: 133 μL autoclaved ddH_2O, 40 μL 5X Maxima RT buffer (Thermo Fisher, EP0753), 20 μL 10 mM dNTPs (NEB, N0447L), 2 μL 1 mM dN-SMRT Oligo (custom from IDT [see sequence below on 20]), 5 μL Klenow Enzyme (NEB, M0210). Prepare before use.

15. cDNA PCR Mix: 88 μL autoclaved ddH_2O, 100 μL Terra PCR Direct Buffer (Takara Biosciences, 639270), 4 μL Terra Polymerase (Takara Biosciences, 639270), 4 μL 100 μM Truseq PCR Handle Primer (custom from IDT [see sequence below on 20]), 4 μL 100 μM SMART PCR Primer (custom from IDT [see sequence below on 20]). Prepare before use.
16. AMPure XP Beads (Beckman Coulter, A63881).
17. Library Prep Reaction Mix: 10 μL Nextera TD Buffer (Illumina, FC-131-1096), 5uL Amplicon Tagmentation Enzyme (Illumina, FC-131-1096), add a total of 600 pg cDNA from the cDNA synthesis step, adjust the total volume to 20 μL with autoclaved ddH_2O. Prepare before use.
18. Nextera PCR Master Mix: 15 μL Nextera PCR mix (Illumina, FC-131-1096), 8uL autoclaved ddH_2O, 1 μL 10 μM P5-Truseq PCR Hybrid Oligo (custom from IDT [see sequence below on 20]), 1 μL 10 μM Nextera N70X oligo (Illumina, FC-131-2001).
19. Sequencing Kit: NextSeq2000 P3 (100 cycle) flow cells (Illumina, 20040559).
20. Template Switch Oligo: AAGCAGTGGTATCAACGCAGAG TGAATrG+GrG.
    Truseq PCR Handle Primer: CTACACGACGCTCTTCCG ATCT.
    SMART PCR Primer: AAGCAGTGGTATCAACGCAGAGT.
    dN-SMRT Oligo: AAGCAGTGGTATCAACGCAGAGTGA NNNGGNNNB,
    P5-Truseq PCR Hybrid Oligo: AATGATACGGCGACCACC GAGATCTACACTCTTTCCCTACACGACGCTCTTCCGA TCT.

3 Methods

3.1 Tissue Dissection and Embedding

1. Before experiment, inspect the pucks under stereomicroscope. Only pucks without obvious space between beads will be used for experiments.
2. Pre-chill HBSS and O.C.T. on ice (over 10 min).
3. Inject the mice intraperitoneally with urethane (10 μL/g × body weight). Under full anesthesia, decapitate the mice, remove the brains from the skull, and rinse brains with ice-cold HBSS to remove blood (*see* **Note 1**).
4. Separate the olfactory bulbs from the brain using a scalpel by a vertical cut along the dorsal-ventral axis slightly behind the OBs. Transfer the tissues into pre-cooled O.C.T. in a small

petri dish (351007, Falcon® 60 mm × 15 mm, Corning) to remove liquid and then transfer the tissue to embedding molds (4566, Tissue-Tek Cryonold, Sakura).

5. Embed the OBs with pre-chilled O.C.T., and adjust their orientation under a stereomicroscope to ensure that the rostral part of the OBs points downward. Flash freeze at −70 °C (HistoChill, Novec™ 7000) (*see* **Note 2**). Tissues can be kept at −70 °C for up to 1 month. Stored tissues need to be wrapped with aluminum foil and kept in sealed plastic bags to prevent dehydrate.

3.2 Tissue Sectioning

1. On the day of tissue sectioning, remove the tissue blocks from −70 °C storage, and warm it inside a Cryostat microtome (CryoStar, NX70) to approximately −20 °C.
2. Mount the block on the cutting stage and section it at 10 μm thickness. Temperature setting: Chamber Temperature: −12 °C, Object Temperature: −10 °C (temperatures need to be adjusted based on sample conditions).
3. Ensure slices are flat, no tear or damage on it. Place slices on the pucks (*see* **Note 3**). Collect slices around 1.6 mm from the anterior OB boundary. Adjacent slices should be also collected on normal slides for H&E and DAPI staining to check for tissue integrity (Fig. 1a–c).
4. Immediately after the tissues are collected on the pucks, immerse the puck in 200 μL hybridization buffer for approximately 30 min at room temperature to facilitate the binding of tissue mRNA to the spatially barcoded beads of the puck (Fig. 1d; **Note 4**).

3.3 Library Preparation

1. After hybridization, transfer the pucks into 200 μL Reverse Transcription Solution, incubate for 30 min at room temperature followed by 1.5 h at 52 °C. This reverse transcription step allows the first strand cDNA to be synthesized from RNA molecules captured on the beads.
2. After reverse transcription, digest the tissue on the pucks by adding 200 μL 2x Tissue Digestion Buffer directly into Reserve Transcription Solution and incubating at 37 °C for 30 min (Fig. 1d).
3. Add 200 μL of Wash Buffer following the digestion. Pipetted up and down several times to release the beads from the coverslip. Once the beads have been released, remove the coverslip with forceps (Fig. 1d; *see* **Note 5**).
4. Centrifuge the tubes under 3000 RCF for 3 min, discard the supernatant, and resuspend the precipitated beads with 200 μL Wash Buffer.
5. Repeat step 4 twice to remove residual enzymes and dNTPs.

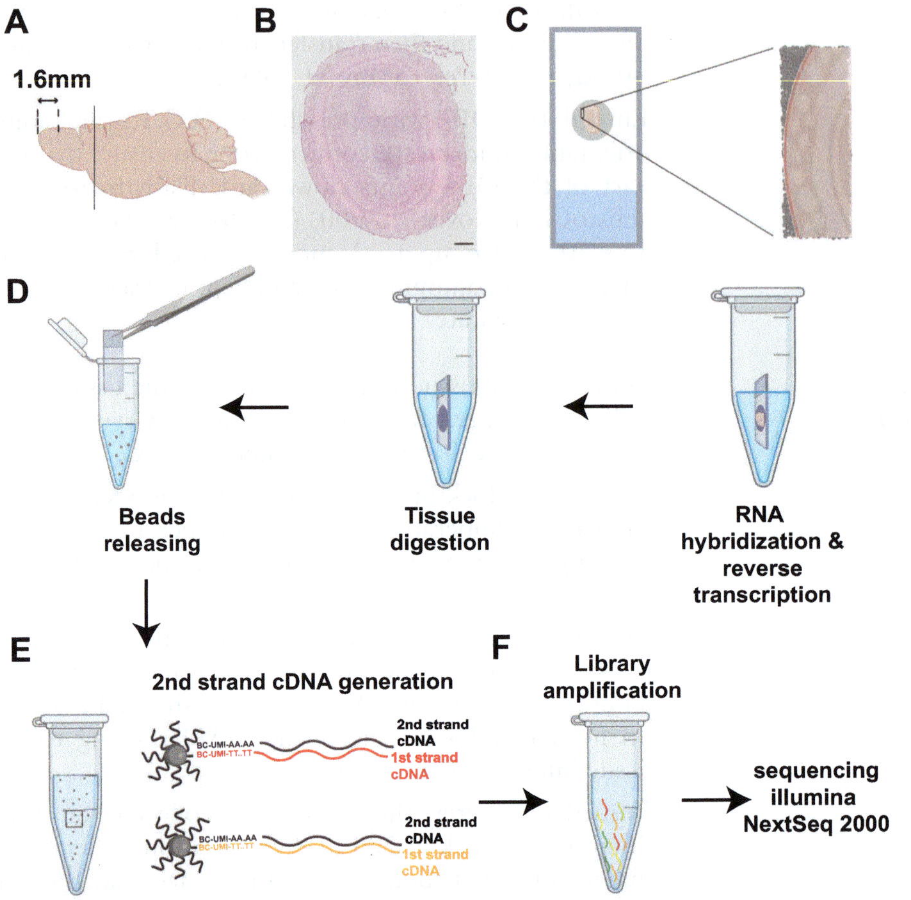

Fig. 1 Illustration of slide-seq procedure (**a**) The mouse brain is cut behind OB (black line) to remove excess tissue. Coronal sections are collected at the 1.6 mm from the anterior edge of olfactory bulb. (**b**) H&E staining showing the morphology of the section. Only slices from tissues without damage or malformation are used for downstream experiments. (**c**) Illustration of placement of the tissue section on the puck. Magnified view illustrates how the tissue is laid on top of the beads. (**d**) Illustration of the pucks with section immersed in hybridization buffer for mRNA capturing, tissue digestion, and beads releasing. (**e**) Process for cDNA synthesis. (**f**) Process for library amplification and sequencing. (Arrows from **c** to **f** indicate experimental flow. Scale bar: 200 μm in panel (**b**))

6. After the third centrifugation step, add 200 μL 10 mM Tris–HCl (pH 8.0), and centrifuge the tube at 3000 RCF for 3 min. Remove the supernatant.
7. Resuspend the samples with Exonuclease I Solution, and incubate for 50 min at 37 °C to degrade free-floating single-strand DNA, this step will reduce background.
8. Wash the beads using 200 μL Wash Buffer, centrifuge for 3 min at 3000 RCF, removing the supernatant, and resuspending the beads. Repeat once.

9. After the last wash, resuspend the beads with 0.1 N NaOH, and incubate for 5 min at room temperature. NaOH incubation would denature the RNA-DNA complex and release the RNA molecules.
10. Wash twice with 200 μL Wash Buffer as in Step 8 (*see* **Note 6**).
11. Resuspend the beads in 200 μL TE buffer, pellet down, remove the supernatant, resuspend them in 200 μL Second Strand Mix, and incubate for 1 h at 37 °C. This step generates second strand cDNA from the first strand on the beads (Fig. 1e).
12. Wash the beads three times with 200 μL Wash Buffer as in Step 8. Perform a final wash in 200 μL of autoclaved ddH_2O, pellet down, remove the supernatant, and resuspend them in cDNA PCR Mix. Transfer the mix into PCR tubes for PCR (*see* **Note 7**).
13. cDNA was amplified by PCR using the following program:

    98 °C 3 min

    Four cycles of

    98 °C, 20 s

    65 °C, 45 s

    72 °C, 3 min

    Nine cycles of

    98 °C, 20 sec

    67 °C, 20 sec

    72 °C, 3 min

    72 °C, 5 min

    4 °C, forever
14. Purify the PCR products with 0.6X AMPure XP Beads twice, resuspend in 20 μL autoclaved ddH_2O, and check for quality and quantity using the Bioanalyzer (Agilent) and Qubit Fluorometer (Thermo Fisher). Expected cDNA concentration should be above 0.15 ng/μL. The size of cDNA is organism-dependent, typically between 1000 and 2000 bp.
15. Perform library preparation using the Nextera XT kit (Illumina, FC-131-1096) reagents. Incubate 600 pg of cDNA with the Library Prep Reaction Mixes at 55 °C for 5 min. After incubation, add 5 μL of Neutralization Buffer (Illumina, FC-131-1096), mix with pipetting, then incubate at room temperature for 5 min. Add Nextera PCR MasterMix to the solution and mix by pipetting (*see* **Note 8**).
16. Perform library amplification by PCR using the following program (Fig. 1f):

    72 °C 3 min

    95 °C, 30 s

12 cycles of
95 °C, 10 s
55 °C, 30 s
72 °C, 30 s
72 °C, 5 min
10 °C, forever

17. Purify the PCR product with 0.6X AMPure XP Beads once, resuspend in 10 μL autoclaved ddH_2O, and check for quality and quantity using the Bioanalyzer (Agilent) and Qubit Fluorometer (Thermo Fisher). Libraries are normally above 3 ng/ μL in concentration and between 400 and 700 bp in length.

3.4 Sequencing

Perform sequencing. We used a P3 flow cell on an Illumina NextSeq 2000 instrument controlled by the NextSeq 2000 1.4.0.39521 software with the following paired read length: 42 bp Read1, 8 bp i7 Index, and 60 bp Read2. Illumina Primary Analysis version NextSeq2K RTA 3.9.2 and Secondary Analysis version bcl2fastq2 v2.20 were run to demultiplex reads for all libraries and generate FASTQ files (Fig. 1f).

3.5 Sequencing Data Analysis

Single-cell RNA-seq data can be leveraged to enhance cell clustering. Before we divide the analysis into two parts.

scRNA-Seq Data Analysis

1. We aligned scRNA-seq reads to mm10 mouse genome reference from UCSC using CellRanger (v4.0.0; 10X Genomics). Annotation was from Ensembl 102.
2. We made a cutoff to maintain cells with 2000–5000 genes and less than 5% mitochondrial counts for downstream analysis.
3. We used DoubletFinder (v2.0.03) [39] to remove doublets from each individual dataset assuming a 7.5% doublet formation rate.
4. We used Seurat SCTransform V2 to process each individual sample and merge them into a single Seurat object. We then performed PCA dimensional reduction and ran FindClusters using 50 PCs with 0.3 resolution.
5. We annotated the clusters with marker genes expression patterns: mitral/tufted cell, Cdhr1, Uchl1, and Emoes; GABAergic interneurons, Gad1, Gad2, and Meis2; oligodendrocytes, Olig2 and Cspg4; astrocytes, Slc1a3 and Gfap; microglia, Ctss and Hexb; olfactory ensheathing cells (OECs), Plp1 and Npy; meninges, Slc6a13 and Cxcl12; pericyte, Myl9; endothelial cells, Pecam1 and Cd34.

Slide-Seq Data Analysis

1. We aligned sequencing reads to mm10 mouse genome reference from UCSC using CellRanger (v4.0.0; 10X Genomics). Annotation was from Ensembl 102. Only beads with barcode mismatch <= 1 and UMI counts > = 10 were kept for future analysis.
2. After generating the expression matrix, we assigned each bead to a location on the puck according to the original spatial barcode information. Files containing the expression matrix and coordinate location were exported for further analysis.
3. Using prior knowledge regarding the anatomical structure, we used the R package gatepoints to manually select the cells in the olfactory bulb. Other spurious cells around the periphery were discarded from further analysis (Fig. 2a). Most beads can detect

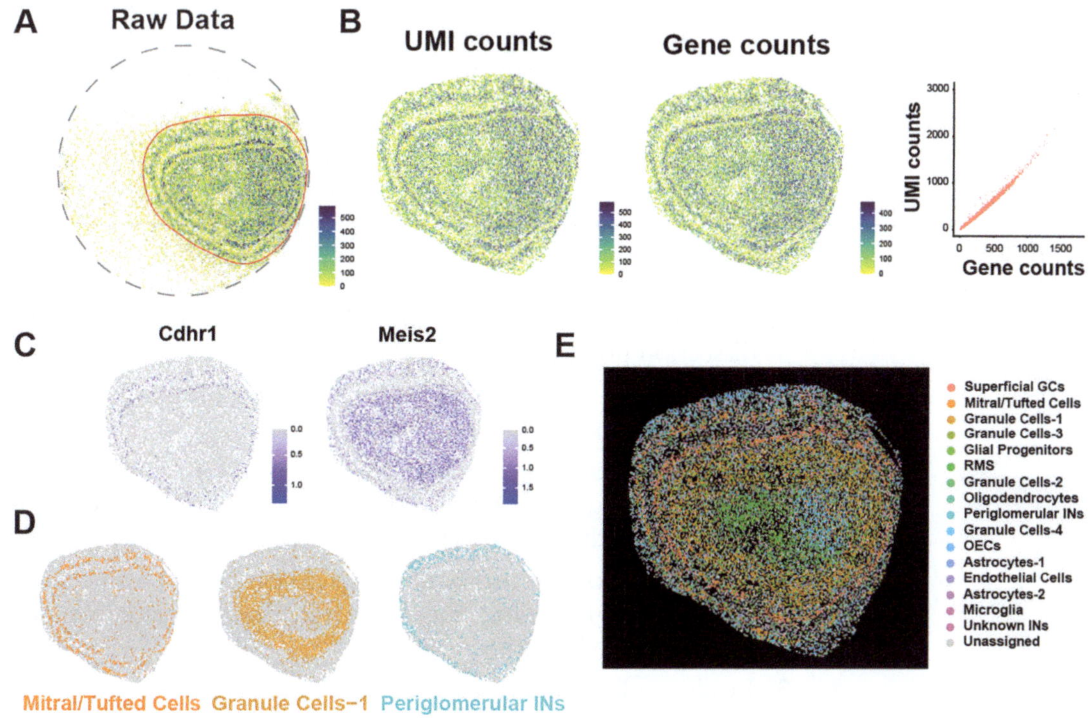

Fig. 2 P7 OB slide-seq result revealed distinguished cell types. (**a**) Total unique molecule index (UMI) count mapped onto the puck. Tissue area was circle (red lined area) to remove signals in the background. (**b**) Heatmaps showing the total UMI (left) and gene (right) counts mapped to the beads. Scatter plot between UMI counts and gene counts indicates relative low depth of slide-seq. (**c**) Neuronal markers detected by slide-seq data are found in the expected locations. Cdhr1 is located to the mitral/tufted cell layer. Meis2 is located to the inner plexiform layer where GABAergic interneurons reside. (**d**, **e**) Multiple cell types are identified based on single-cell cluster features and located in the section based on the spatial information. Cell types are marked based on marker gene expression and are color coded. Abbreviations: *GC* granule cell, *RMS* rostral migratory stream, *IN* interneuron, *OEC* olfactory ensheathing cell

100–580 UMIs and 75–450 genes with around 1.5 UMIs/genes ratio (Fig. 2b).

4. We used Seurat functions FindTransferAnchors and TransferData to transfer cluster labels in the scRNA-seq data to the Slide-Seq data [40]. For each individual slide-seq pixel (bead), the probability that it belongs to the same cell type as the single-cell clusters is calculated, with probabilities summing up to 1 across all cell types. The single-cell cluster with the highest probability was used as the assigned label for each pixel. If no individual single-cell cluster receives above a 0.25 probability, the pixel is labeled as "Unassigned" (Fig. 2e).
5. We annotate the cluster using a combination of marker gene expression patterns and spatial patterns of single-cell clusters across the tissue. Using known marker genes of specific cell types, single-cell cluster annotations were assigned and transferred over to the slide-seq data. For clusters with no strong known marker genes, previous anatomical knowledge along with the spatial pattern of the slide-seq pixels in the olfactory bulb of a given cluster was used to inform cluster annotations (Fig. 2c, d, and e).

4 Notes

1. Dissection for each animal should be finished in 2–3 min. All dissection process should be performed on ice.
2. Fresh tissues with O.C.T. need to be frozen rapidly for preventing crystals formation.
3. Slices need to be placed in the middle of the puck, where the beads are (Fig. 1c). Double confirm slices are fully attached to the beads without bubbles.
4. The timing for this incubation step is kept consistent between all samples, following the Broad Institute's recommended 15–30 min hybridization time.
5. Beads can be visually observed dislocating from the puck.
6. Insufficient wash may result in high background for sequencing data.
7. Each 200 μL sample is split into two PCR tubes prior to cDNA amplification.
8. The library preparation described is performed according to manufacturer's directions for the Nextera XT kit (Illumina, FC-131-1096), modifying the starting input of material to 600 pg of cDNA and using a specific P5-Truseq PCR hybrid oligo in place of the Nextera XT i5 adapter.

Acknowledgments

We thank Dr. Fei Chen and Mr. Evan Murray at Broad Institute for providing the pre-sequenced pucks. We thank Lab Animal Service Facility, Histology, Sequencing, and Microscopy Center of Stowers Institute for their technical assistance. We also thank Yu lab members for their insightful discussions. This work was supported by funding from NIH (R01DC016696 and R01DC014701) and Stowers Institute for Medical Research to C.R.Y.

Author Contribution C.R.Y. and A.F. conceived the project. A.F. and C.R.Y. designed the experiments. M.T. managed mouse colonies. A.F. dissected tissues. S.M. embedded tissues, captured slices onto pucks and slides, and performed H&E staining for adjacent slices, Y.W. supervised histology process. C.M. imaged H&E and DAPI stained slices. S.M. supervised slice imaging. K.P. performed all library preparation steps, A.P. supervised library preparation and contacted the Broad Institute. M.P. performed sequencing for the library. J.R. ran the CellRanger pipeline. A.P. and A.F. analyzed slide-seq data. H.L. supervised bioinformatics analysis. A.F. made all figs. C.R.Y., A.F., K.P., and A.P. wrote the paper.

References

1. Fletcher RB, Das D, Gadye L, Street KN, Baudhuin A, Wagner A, Cole MB, Flores Q, Choi YG, Yosef N, Purdom E, Dudoit S, Risso D, Ngai J (2017) Deconstructing olfactory stem cell trajectories at single-cell resolution. Cell Stem Cell 20(6):817–830 e818. https://doi.org/10.1016/j.stem.2017.04.003
2. Tepe B, Hill MC, Pekarek BT, Hunt PJ, Martin TJ, Martin JF, Arenkiel BR (2018) Single-cell RNA-Seq of mouse olfactory bulb reveals cellular heterogeneity and activity-dependent molecular census of adult-born neurons. Cell Rep 25(10):2689–2703 e2683. https://doi.org/10.1016/j.celrep.2018.11.034
3. Wu Y, Ma L, Duyck K, Long CC, Moran A, Scheerer H, Blanck J, Peak A, Box A, Perera A, Yu CR (2018) A population of navigator neurons is essential for olfactory map formation during the critical period. Neuron 100(5): 1066–1082. e1066. https://doi.org/10.1016/j.neuron.2018.09.051
4. Hanchate NK, Kondoh K, Lu Z, Kuang D, Ye X, Qiu X, Pachter L, Trapnell C, Buck LB (2015) Single-cell transcriptomics reveals receptor transformations during olfactory neurogenesis. Science 350(6265):1251–1255. https://doi.org/10.1126/science.aad2456
5. Tsukahara T, Brann DH, Pashkovski SL, Guitchounts G, Bozza T, Datta SR (2021) A transcriptional rheostat couples past activity to future sensory responses. Cell 184(26): 6326–6343 e6332. https://doi.org/10.1016/j.cell.2021.11.022
6. Vihani A, Hu XS, Gundala S, Koyama S, Block E, Matsunami H (2020) Semiochemical responsive olfactory sensory neurons are sexually dimorphic and plastic. eLife 9:e54501. https://doi.org/10.7554/eLife.54501
7. Horgue LF, Assens A, Fodoulian L, Marconi L, Tuberosa J, Haider A, Boillat M, Carleton A, Rodriguez I (2022) Transcriptional adaptation of olfactory sensory neurons to GPCR identity and activity. Nat Commun 13(1):2929. https://doi.org/10.1038/s41467-022-30,511-4
8. Duyck K, DuTell V, Ma L, Paulson A, Yu CR (2017) Pronounced strain-specific chemosensory receptor gene expression in the mouse vomeronasal organ. BMC Genomics 18(1): 965. https://doi.org/10.1186/s12864-017-4364-4

9. Wang Y, Jiang H, Yang L (2020) Transcriptome analysis of zebrafish olfactory epithelium reveal sexual differences in odorant detection. Genes 11(6):592. https://doi.org/10.3390/genes11060592
10. Tang F, Barbacioru C, Wang Y, Nordman E, Lee C, Xu N, Wang X, Bodeau J, Tuch BB, Siddiqui A, Lao K, Surani MA (2009) mRNA-Seq whole-transcriptome analysis of a single cell. Nat Methods 6(5):377–382. https://doi.org/10.1038/nmeth.1315
11. Nawy T (2014) Single-cell sequencing. Nat Methods 11(1):18. https://doi.org/10.1038/nmeth.2771
12. Shapiro E, Biezuner T, Linnarsson S (2013) Single-cell sequencing-based technologies will revolutionize whole-organism science. Nat Rev Genet 14(9):618–630. https://doi.org/10.1038/nrg3542
13. Chen KH, Boettiger AN, Moffitt JR, Wang S, Zhuang X (2015) RNA imaging. Spatially resolved, highly multiplexed RNA profiling in single cells. Science 348(6233):aaa6090. https://doi.org/10.1126/science.aaa6090
14. Moffitt JR, Hao J, Wang G, Chen KH, Babcock HP, Zhuang X (2016) High-throughput single-cell gene-expression profiling with multiplexed error-robust fluorescence in situ hybridization. Proc Natl Acad Sci USA 113(39):11046–11051. https://doi.org/10.1073/pnas.1612826113
15. Moffitt JR, Hao J, Bambah-Mukku D, Lu T, Dulac C, Zhuang X (2016) High-performance multiplexed fluorescence in situ hybridization in culture and tissue with matrix imprinting and clearing. Proc Natl Acad Sci USA 113(50):14456–14461. https://doi.org/10.1073/pnas.1617699113
16. Guilliams M, Bonnardel J, Haest B, Vanderborght B, Wagner C, Remmerie A, Bujko A, Martens L, Thone T, Browaeys R, De Ponti FF, Vanneste B, Zwicker C, Svedberg FR, Vanhalewyn T, Goncalves A, Lippens S, Devriendt B, Cox E, Ferrero G, Wittamer V, Willaert A, Kaptein SJF, Neyts J, Dallmeier K, Geldhof P, Casaert S, Deplancke B, Ten Dijke P, Hoorens A, Vanlander A, Berrevoet F, Van Nieuwenhove Y, Saeys Y, Saelens W, Van Vlierberghe H, Devisscher L, Scott CL (2022) Spatial proteogenomics reveals distinct and evolutionarily conserved hepatic macrophage niches. Cell 185(2):379–396 e338. https://doi.org/10.1016/j.cell.2021.12.018
17. Lee JH, Daugharthy ER, Scheiman J, Kalhor R, Yang JL, Ferrante TC, Terry R, Jeanty SS, Li C, Amamoto R, Peters DT, Turczyk BM, Marblestone AH, Inverso SA, Bernard A, Mali P, Rios X, Aach J, Church GM (2014) Highly multiplexed subcellular RNA sequencing in situ. Science 343(6177):1360–1363. https://doi.org/10.1126/science.1250212
18. Lee JH, Daugharthy ER, Scheiman J, Kalhor R, Ferrante TC, Terry R, Turczyk BM, Yang JL, Lee HS, Aach J, Zhang K, Church GM (2015) Fluorescent in situ sequencing (FISSEQ) of RNA for gene expression profiling in intact cells and tissues. Nat Protoc 10(3):442–458. https://doi.org/10.1038/nprot.2014.191
19. Eng CL, Lawson M, Zhu Q, Dries R, Koulena N, Takei Y, Yun J, Cronin C, Karp C, Yuan GC, Cai L (2019) Transcriptome-scale super-resolved imaging in tissues by RNA seqFISH. Nature 568(7751):235–239. https://doi.org/10.1038/s41586-019-1049-y
20. Wang X, Allen WE, Wright MA, Sylwestrak EL, Samusik N, Vesuna S, Evans K, Liu C, Ramakrishnan C, Liu J, Nolan GP, Bava FA, Deisseroth K (2018) Three-dimensional intact-tissue sequencing of single-cell transcriptional states. Science 361(6400):eaat5691. https://doi.org/10.1126/science.aat5691
21. Goltsev Y, Samusik N, Kennedy-Darling J, Bhate S, Hale M, Vazquez G, Black S, Nolan GP (2018) Deep profiling of mouse splenic architecture with CODEX multiplexed imaging. Cell 174(4):968–981 e915. https://doi.org/10.1016/j.cell.2018.07.010
22. Lein E, Borm LE, Linnarsson S (2017) The promise of spatial transcriptomics for neuroscience in the era of molecular cell typing. Science 358(6359):64–69. https://doi.org/10.1126/science.aan6827
23. Stahl PL, Salmen F, Vickovic S, Lundmark A, Navarro JF, Magnusson J, Giacomello S, Asp M, Westholm JO, Huss M, Mollbrink A, Linnarsson S, Codeluppi S, Borg A, Ponten F, Costea PI, Sahlen P, Mulder J, Bergmann O, Lundeberg J, Frisen J (2016) Visualization and analysis of gene expression in tissue sections by spatial transcriptomics. Science 353(6294):78–82. https://doi.org/10.1126/science.aaf2403
24. Chen A, Liao S, Cheng M, Ma K, Wu L, Lai Y, Qiu X, Yang J, Xu J, Hao S, Wang X, Lu H, Chen X, Liu X, Huang X, Li Z, Hong Y, Jiang Y, Peng J, Liu S, Shen M, Liu C, Li Q, Yuan Y, Wei X, Zheng H, Feng W, Wang Z, Liu Y, Wang Z, Yang Y, Xiang H, Han L, Qin B, Guo P, Lai G, Munoz-Canoves P, Maxwell PH, Thiery JP, Wu QF, Zhao F, Chen B, Li M, Dai X, Wang S, Kuang H, Hui J, Wang L, Fei JF, Wang O, Wei X, Lu H, Wang B, Liu S,

Gu Y, Ni M, Zhang W, Mu F, Yin Y, Yang H, Lisby M, Cornall RJ, Mulder J, Uhlen M, Esteban MA, Li Y, Liu L, Xu X, Wang J (2022) Spatiotemporal transcriptomic atlas of mouse organogenesis using DNA nanoball-patterned arrays. Cell 185(10):1777–1792. e1721. https://doi.org/10.1016/j.cell.2022.04.003

25. Mombaerts P (2006) Axonal wiring in the mouse olfactory system. Annu Rev Cell Dev Biol 22:713–737. https://doi.org/10.1146/annurev.cellbio.21.012804.093915

26. Sakano H (2020) Developmental regulation of olfactory circuit formation in mice. Develop Growth Differ 62(4):199–213. https://doi.org/10.1111/dgd.12657

27. Sakano H (2010) Neural map formation in the mouse olfactory system. Neuron 67(4): 530–542. https://doi.org/10.1016/j.neuron.2010.07.003

28. Ma L, Wu Y, Qiu Q, Scheerer H, Moran A, Yu CR (2014) A developmental switch of axon targeting in the continuously regenerating mouse olfactory system. Science 344(6180): 194–197. https://doi.org/10.1126/science.1248805

29. Tsai L, Barnea G (2014) A critical period defined by axon-targeting mechanisms in the murine olfactory bulb. Science 344(6180): 197–200. https://doi.org/10.1126/science.1248806

30. Cheetham CEJ, Park U, Belluscio L (2016) Rapid and continuous activity-dependent plasticity of olfactory sensory input. Nat Commun 7:10729. https://doi.org/10.1038/ncomms10729

31. Singh DN, Nathaniel EJ (1977) Postnatal development of mitral cell perikaryon in the olfactory bulb of the rat. A light and ultrastructural study. Anat Rec 189(3):413–431. https://doi.org/10.1002/ar.1091890303

32. Lin DM, Wang F, Lowe G, Gold GH, Axel R, Ngai J, Brunet L (2000) Formation of precise connections in the olfactory bulb occurs in the absence of odorant-evoked neuronal activity. Neuron 26(1):69–80. https://doi.org/10.1016/s0896-6273(00)81139-3

33. Cao L, Dhilla A, Mukai J, Blazeski R, Lodovichi C, Mason CA, Gogos JA (2007) Genetic modulation of BDNF signaling affects the outcome of axonal competition in vivo. Curr Biol 17(11):911–921. https://doi.org/10.1016/j.cub.2007.04.040

34. Batista-Brito R, Close J, Machold R, Fishell G (2008) The distinct temporal origins of olfactory bulb interneuron subtypes. J Neurosci 28(15):3966–3975. https://doi.org/10.1523/jneurosci.5625-07.2008

35. Angelova A, Tiveron MC, Cremer H, Beclin C (2018) Neuronal subtype generation during postnatal olfactory bulb neurogenesis. J Exp Neurosci 12:1179069518755670. https://doi.org/10.1177/1179069518755670

36. Rodriques SG, Stickels RR, Goeva A, Martin CA, Murray E, Vanderburg CR, Welch J, Chen LM, Chen F, Macosko EZ (2019) Slide-seq: a scalable technology for measuring genome-wide expression at high spatial resolution. Science 363(6434):1463–1467. https://doi.org/10.1126/science.aaw1219

37. Stickels RR, Murray E, Kumar P, Li J, Marshall JL, Di Bella DJ, Arlotta P, Macosko EZ, Chen F (2021) Highly sensitive spatial transcriptomics at near-cellular resolution with slide-seqV2. Nat Biotechnol 39(3):313–319. https://doi.org/10.1038/s41587-020-0739-1

38. Wu Y, Ma L, Qiu Q, Xu W, Misra A, Duyck K, Blanck J, Scott AR, Chen S, Hassan H, Corbin TJ, Moran A, Hall K, Li H, Perera A, Yu CR (2022) Molecular control of circuit plasticity and the permanence of imprinted odor memory. bioRxiv:2022.2003.2029.486284. https://doi.org/10.1101/2022.03.29.486284

39. McGinnis CS, Murrow LM, Gartner ZJ (2019) DoubletFinder: doublet detection in single-cell RNA sequencing data using artificial nearest neighbors. Cell Syst 8(4):329–337 e324. https://doi.org/10.1016/j.cels.2019.03.003

40. Hao Y, Hao S, Andersen-Nissen E, Mauck WM, Zheng S, Butler A, Lee MJ, Wilk AJ, Darby C, Zager M, Hoffman P, Stoeckius M, Papalexi E, Mimitou EP, Jain J, Srivastava A, Stuart T, Fleming LM, Yeung B, Rogers AJ, JM ME, Blish CA, Gottardo R, Smibert P, Satija R (2021) Integrated analysis of multimodal single-cell data. Cell 184(13): 3573–3587 e3529. https://doi.org/10.1016/j.cell.2021.04.048

Chapter 14

Dense and Sparse Labelling of Mitral Cells by Oral and Intraperitoneal Routes of Tamoxifen Administration

Xiaochen Fu, Yu-Pei Huang, Sander Lindeman, Adam Mago, and Izumi Fukunaga

Abstract

Cell type-specific labelling and manipulation using Cre-driver lines have become integral to analyses of neuronal circuits in the brain. To study how mitral cells of the olfactory bulb process olfactory information and how they contribute to behavior, an inducible Cre-driver line, Lbhd2-CreER^{T2}, can be used. In this chapter, we describe two methods for administering tamoxifen. The first method achieves a dense recombination pattern using tamoxifen-containing food, while the second method involving an intraperitoneal injection is suited for sparse labelling.

Key words Cre-ER^{T2}, Olfactory bulb, Tamoxifen, Cell types, Mitral cells

1 Introduction

Distinguishing different cell types is a fundamental aspect of experiments aimed to understand how circuits in the brain work [1, 2]. A wide range of driver lines, such as those that express Cre recombinase in specific cell types, have become integral to such investigations [3, 4]. In the mammalian olfactory system, complex information processing starts in the olfactory bulb, whose output is conveyed by mitral cells and tufted cells [5, 6]. Mitral cell-selective labelling and manipulation have recently become possible with the generation of Lbhd2-CreER^{T2} line [7].

Cre-ER^{T2} is an inducible form of Cre recombinase, where the Cre is bound to a modified human estrogen receptor that carries triple mutations [8]. This modified receptor is insensitive to 17β-estradiol but binds a metabolite of tamoxifen, 4-hydroxytamoxifen, to induce Cre recombinase activity. Tamoxifen delivery was initially achieved by intraperitoneal injections and oral gavage [9, 10]. Later, a less intrusive method of administration

Bradley J. Goldstein and Hiroaki Matsunami (eds.), *The Olfactory System*, Methods in Molecular Biology, vol. 2710, https://doi.org/10.1007/978-1-0716-3425-7_14,

involving an oral route with food containing tamoxifen or tamoxifen citrate was introduced and has been used routinely [11–14].

The exact tamoxifen administration protocol for achieving the desired recombination pattern depends on the mouse model, the purpose of the study, and ethical considerations. Many protocols describe the administration in adult mice [11–13]. For mitral cell-selective recombination using the Lbhd2-CreER^{T2} line, tamoxifen administration around P21 was found to be desirable [7]. Even when using the same transgenic line, however, some experiments require a dense recombination pattern, for example, when exhaustive characterization or perturbation of mitral cell population is required. On the other hand, other experiments may require a sparse recombination pattern, for example, when studying the morphology or the physiology of single cells or their subcellular compartments in isolation. To achieve a dense recombination pattern where repeated or continuous tamoxifen administration is required, the oral route may be more ethical and comparable compared to a large number of injections. On the other hand, due to the voluntary nature of tamoxifen administration, it isn't easy to control dosage precisely using the food. Thus, an intraperitoneal injection may be preferable when a smaller and specific dose is needed.

In this protocol, we describe two protocols for tamoxifen administration, first, via tamoxifen-containing food leading to a dense recombination pattern in a dose-dependent manner, and, second, an intraperitoneal injection that leads to sparse labelling. When administering tamoxifen via food, previous methods ranged in the durations of exposure between 1 and 2 weeks [11] or sometimes 1–2 months. The protocol described here uses a relatively high tamoxifen content in the food of 2 mg/g [13], which shortens the exposure to 3 days maximum, avoiding prolonged tamoxifen exposure for animals and experimenters. In addition, we describe an optional method to estimate the amount of food consumed by individual mice in a group housing. This method considers individual differences in food consumption rather than assuming equal consumption [13].

2 Materials

Tamoxifen is light-sensitive and should be stored away from light. In addition, because tamoxifen is an estrogen receptor antagonist [15], direct contact should be avoided. Appropriate personal protective equipment should be worn, cages should be clearly labelled, and waste should be properly disposed according to local regulations.

1. *Mice*

21-day-old Lbhd2-CreER^{T2} mice [7] [deposited as C57BL/6 J-Lbhd2em1(cre/ERT2)Fuki/J; strain number 036054 at Jackson Laboratory] crossed with a reporter line (e.g., Ai14 [16]

B6;129S6-Gt(ROSA)26Sor-tm(CAG-tdTomato)Hze/J or Ai95D [17] B6;129S-Gt(ROSA)26Sor-tm95.1(CAG-GCaMP6f)Hze/J). (*see* **Note 1**).

2. *Tamoxifen-containing diet*

Tamoxifen (e.g., Sigma-Aldrich T5648) is mixed with crushed food at a composition of 2 g/kg. A convenient source of tamoxifen diet is a veterinary food vendor, which mixes the tamoxifen and food and supplies them as sterilized pellets (*see* **Note 2**).

1. If ready-made pellets are used, aliquot the tamoxifen-containing pellets in air-tight plastic bags. About 30–50 g will be enough for three to five mice for 3 days.
2. Add desiccators in a light-proof container, then add the aliquoted tamoxifen-containing food. Seal the container and store in a cold room (5 °C) until use.

3. *Tamoxifen solution for injection*

Tamoxifen solution (8 mg/ml in a mixture of ethanol and corn oil at 5%/95%, vol/vol)) should be prepared just before use. To prepare enough tamoxifen solution for a number (n) of mice, calculate the amount of tamoxifen and the volume of solvent required as follows (*see* **Note 3**):

$$\text{Amount of tamoxifen (mg)} = \frac{80 \times \text{average weight (g)} \times \text{number of mice}}{1000}$$

$$\text{Volume of corn oil mixture (ml)} = \frac{\text{Amount of tamoxifen to use (mg)}}{8}$$

The method here describes the preparation of a tamoxifen solution for five mice at postnatal 21 days old (P21), weighing 10 g on average. Due to the solvent's viscosity, enough solution for seven mice (five actual + two spare mice) is prepared:

1. Preheat the oven to 65 °C. Ideally, a small portable shaker is also placed inside.
2. In a 5 ml microtube, weigh 5.6 mg tamoxifen on an analytical balance.
3. Add 35 μl absolute ethanol to the above tamoxifen and mix well.
4. Add 665 μl of corn oil to the above tamoxifen mixture (*see* **Note 4**).
5. Wrap the outer surface of the microtube with an aluminum foil to block light.
6. Heat the tamoxifen mixture at 65 °C on a shaker in the oven for 30 min.
7. Remove from the oven and allow to cool to room temperature.

4. *Glucose saline (makes 25 ml)*

Weigh 0.225 g NaCl and 1.25 g glucose. Dissolve NaCl and glucose in 25 ml ultrapure water. Sterile filter the solution using a sterile syringe and 0.22 μm pore syringe filter.

3 Method

We describe two methods for tamoxifen administrations to achieve mitral cell-selective recombination patterns in Lbhd2-CreER^{T2} mice (Fig. 1). Dense labelling is achieved by the administration through a tamoxifen-containing diet. For sparse labelling, a more reliable method is an intraperitoneal injection of tamoxifen.

3.1 Dense Labelling with Tamoxifen-Containing Chow

3.1.1 Day 1: Replacing the Normal Food with Tamoxifen-Containing Food

1. Enter the weight of each mouse in the cage into the health record (*see* **Note 5**).
2. Take a fresh aliquot of the tamoxifen food (about 30–50 g per cage with five mice). Weigh the initial amount.
3. Remove the existing, normal food from the cage, and replace it with the tamoxifen-containing food pellets (*see* **Note 6**).

3.1.2 Days 2–3: Oral tamoxifen Administration Via Tamoxifen-Containing Diet

1. Weigh each mouse in the cage and note the weight into the health record.
2. Weigh the tamoxifen-containing chow remaining in the cage.
3. If the mouse's weight is above 80% of the weight on Day 1, return the mouse to the same cage.
4. If the mouse's weight is less than 80% of original, the mouse should be put back on the normal diet in a separate cage and supplemented with a subcutaneous injection of glucose saline (0.1–0.2 ml).
5. Repeat steps 1–4 until Day 3, or until 300 mg/kg of tamoxifen has been consumed. For a 10 g mouse, this corresponds to consumption of 1.5 g of the tamoxifen-containing food.

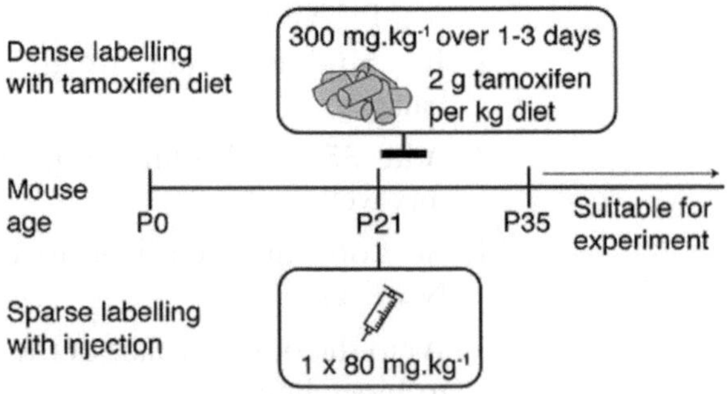

Fig. 1 Timelines of tamoxifen administration. For both methods, administering tamoxifen around P21 gives a good compromise between convenience, the efficiency of recombination, and selectivity

3.1.3 Day 4: Post-administration Monitoring and Determination of tamoxifen Consumed by Group-Housed Mice

1. On Day 4, remove the tamoxifen-containing diet from the cage, and replace it with normal food. The tamoxifen-containing food should be discarded in a sealed bag and according to the local regulation.
2. Monitor the weight of the mice for 2 days after the end of tamoxifen administration.
3. If needed, calculate the amount of tamoxifen consumed by individual mice based on their health record and daily tamoxifen consumption (**steps 4–8**).
4. For group-housed mice, the amount of food consumed each day (d) by each mouse (i) is proportional to the total amount of food consumed each day by all mice in the cage: (Difference in the amount of food remaining : $F^{d-1} - F^{d}$) and inversely proportional to the weight loss $\left(W_i^{d-1} - W_i^{d}\right)$.
5. Weight estimation of each mouse in group housing is done in two steps. First, use the regression below obtained separately from individually housed mice (*see* **Note 7**):

$$T^{d}_{Indiv\_i} = -0.7205 * \left(W_i^{d-1} - W_i^{d}\right) + 2.8057$$

where $T^{d}_{indiv\_i}$ is the amount of food (in grams) individually caged animal i would have consumed on day d and W_i^d is the weight of the animal i on day d.

6. Second, because the relationship between weight loss and food consumed is slightly different when mice are group-housed, the amount of food consumed (T) by individual animal within the group ($group\_i$) on day d is corrected by the total estimate for all mice (j) in the group as follows:

$$T^{d}_{group\_i} = \frac{T^{d}_{Indiv\_i}}{\sum_j T^{d}_{Indiv\_j}} \times \left(F^{d-1} - F^{d}\right)$$

7. The total amount of food each animal consumed over days (T_i, in grams) is obtained by summing the estimated food consumption per day:

$$T_i = \sum_d T^{d}_{group\_i}$$

8. Finally, the tamoxifen dose for animal i (D_i) is expressed in mg/kg as:

$$D_i = \frac{T_i}{W_i^0} \times \text{Tamoxifen content of food (mg/g)} \times 1000$$

where W_i^0 is the original weight (in g) of each animal.

3.1.4 Day 14 Onward: Induced Expression Level Should Be Suitable for Histology or Other Experiments (Fig. 2)

3.2 Sparse Labelling with an Intraperitoneal Injection

3.2.1 Day 1: Intraperitoneal Injection of Tamoxifen

1. Record the weight of each mouse.
2. Prepare the tamoxifen solution (8 mg/ml).
3. Draw the tamoxifen solution into a 1 ml syringe (*see* **Note 8**).
4. For each mouse, note the weight, and inject 1 ul/g of the mouse weight intraperitoneally using a 26G, 1/2 mm needle (*see* **Note 9**).

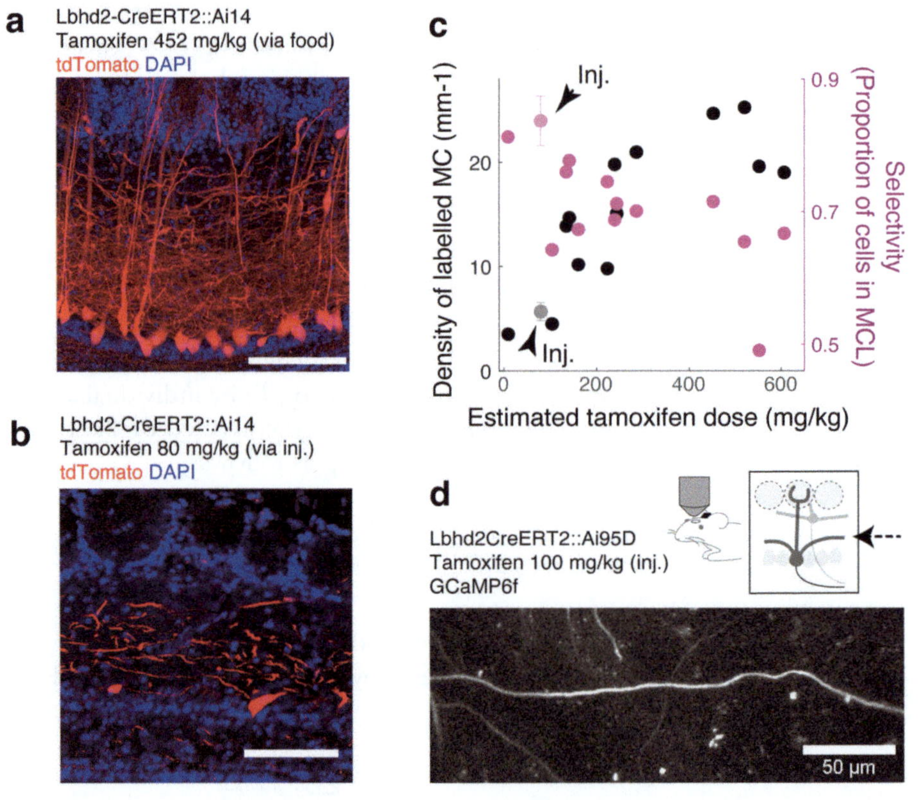

Fig. 2 Recombination pattern in the olfactory bulb using the two tamoxifen administrative methods. (**a**) Dense tdTomato labelling in a Lbhd2-CreER^{T2}::Ai14 mouse 2 weeks after consuming the tamoxifen-containing food (estimated dose, 452.0 mg/kg). Scale bar = 100 mm. (**b**) Sparse tdTomato labelling in a Lbhd2-CreER^{T2}::Ai14 mouse injected intraperitoneally with tamoxifen (1 × 80 mg/kg). Scale bar = 100 mm. (**c**) Quantitative relationships between the density (black) and selectivity (purple) of labelling and the tamoxifen dose, using Lbhd2-CreER^{T2}::Ai14 mice. Dots correspond to individual mice that received tamoxifen-containing food, except for points with error bars, which come from injected animals (n = 4 mice). (**d**) Sparse labelling is useful for studying the physiology of individual mitral cell lateral dendrites in vivo. GCaMP6f fluorescence signals observed with a two-photon microscope, showing the mitral cell dendrites in the external plexiform layer of the olfactory bulb. The Lbhd2-CreER^{T2}::Ai95D mouse received 100 mg/kg tamoxifen via intraperitoneal injection. Scale bar = 50 mm

3.2.2 Day 2: Monitoring

1. Record the weight of each mouse.
2. If the weight is lower than 80% of the original, administer 200 μl glucose saline subcutaneously.

3.2.3 Day 14 Onward: Induced Expression Level Should Be Suitable for Histology or Other Experiments (Fig. 2)

4 Notes

1. The choice of P21 is based on several factors, including a developmental increase in recombination in cell types other than mitral cells and a difficulty in administering tamoxifen to younger mice. A highly mitral cell-selective recombination pattern can be obtained by administering tamoxifen at P7 [7]. However, the administration route is restricted to intraperitoneal injection at this pre-weaning stage.
2. Depending on the vendor, there is a choice of base food and whether tamoxifen or tamoxifen citrate is used. For the base food, a formula with higher sucrose content may lessen animals' aversion. Tamoxifen and tamoxifen citrate are both known to be effective, but for the latter, it should be noted that the tamoxifen content is 66% of its weight. In this protocol, the tamoxifen content in the food was 2 g/kg, to minimize the duration of the exposure. However, a lower content may achieve a more controlled tamoxifen dosage.
3. Corn oil is viscous and sticks to the walls of plastic containers used for preparations, leading to some loss. Therefore, prepare slightly more solution than the strictly required volume.
4. As mentioned in Note 3, the corn oil is viscous. When pipetting this material, aspirate and dispense slowly. Not all oil will be dispensed during the first dispense due to the adherence to the inside wall.
5. At P21, some mice are small (less than 10 g) and have not sufficiently weaned off their mothers. It is best to start the exposure to tamoxifen-containing food 2 days after they are weaned to ensure that the young mice are self-sufficient.
6. Clear communication with the animal caretakers is desirable. Cages with tamoxifen-containing food should be suitably labelled.

7. The regression was obtained in a separate study, where the weight loss and the food consumed of individually house mice were monitored. There was a clear negative correlation between how much animals lost weight per day and the amount of food they ate per day.
8. Viscous materials like corn oil are difficult to aspirate through needles. To avoid bubble formations, fill the syringe without the needle.
9. Injection should be shallow and at an angle to avoid damaging the intestines. Use short needles to estimate the injection depth. After injection, there may be some leakage. The leakage is minimized by avoiding injection of air bubbles.

References

1. Fishell G, Heintz N (2013) Neuron 80(3): 602–612. https://doi.org/10.1016/j.neuron.2013.10.035
2. Zeng H, Sanes JR (2017) Nat Rev Neurosci 18(9):530–546. https://doi.org/10.1038/nrn.2017.85
3. Madisen, L., T. Mao, H. Koch, J.-m. Zhuo, A. Berenyi, S. Fujisawa, Y.-W.A. Hsu, A.J. Garcia, X. Gu, S. Zanella, J. Kidney, H. Gu, Y. Mao, B.M. Hooks, E.S. Boyden, G. Buzsáki, J.M. Ramirez, A.R. Jones, K. Svoboda, X. Han, E.E. Turner, and H. Zeng, Nat Neurosci, (2012. A toolbox of Cre-dependent optogenetic transgenic mice for light-induced activation and silencing. Nat Neurosci 15, 793–802. https://doi.org/10.1038/nn.3078
4. Daigle TL, Madisen L, Hage TA, Valley MT, Knoblich U, Larsen RS, Takeno MM, Huang L, Gu H, Larsen R, Mills M, Bosma-Moody A, Siverts LA, Walker M, Graybuck LT, Yao Z, Fong O, Nguyen TN, Garren E, Lenz GH, Chavarha M, Pendergraft J, Harrington J, Hirokawa KE, Harris JA, Nicovich PR, McGraw MJ, Ollerenshaw DR, Smith KA, Baker CA, Ting JT, Sunkin SM, Lecoq J, Lin MZ, Boyden ES, Murphy GJ, da Costa NM, Waters J, Li L, Tasic B, Zeng H (2018) A suite of transgenic driver and reporter mouse lines with enhanced brain-cell-type targeting and functionality. Cell 174(2):465–480.e22. https://doi.org/10.1016/j.cell.2018.06.035
5. Shepherd GM, Chen WR, Greer CA (2004) Olfactory bulb. In: The synaptic organization of the brain. Oxford University Press, Oxford
6. Mori K, Kishi K, Ojima H (1983) Distribution of dendrites of mitral, displaced mitral, tufted, and granule cells in the rabbit olfactory bulb. J Comp Neurol 219(3):339–355. https://doi.org/10.1002/cne.902190308
7. Koldaeva A, Zhang C, Huang Y-P, Reinert JK, Mizuno S, Sugiyama F, Takahashi S, Soliman T, Matsunami H, Fukunaga I (2021) Generation and characterization of a cell type-specific, inducible Cre-driver line to study olfactory processing. J Neurosci 41(30):6449. https://doi.org/10.1523/jneurosci.3076-20.2021
8. Feil R, Wagner J, Metzger D, Chambon P (1997) Regulation of Cre recombinase activity by mutated estrogen receptor ligand-binding domains. Biochem Biophys Res Commun 237(3):752–757. https://doi.org/10.1006/bbrc.1997.7124
9. Donocoff RS, Teteloshvili N, Chung H, Shoulson R, Creusot RJ (2020) Optimization of tamoxifen-induced Cre activity and its effect on immune cell populations. Sci Rep 10(1): 15244. https://doi.org/10.1038/s41598-020-72179-0
10. Whitfield J, Littlewood T, Soucek L (2015) Tamoxifen administration to mice. Cold Spring Harb Protoc 2015(3):pdb-prot077966
11. Andersson KB, Winer LH, Mørk HK, Molkentin JD, Jaisser F (2010) Tamoxifen administration routes and dosage for inducible Cre-mediated gene disruption in mouse hearts. Transgenic Res 19(4):715–725. https://doi.org/10.1007/s11248-009-9342-4
12. Kiermayer, C., M. Conrad, M. Schneider, J. Schmidt, And M. Brielmeier, Optimization of spatiotemporal gene inactivation in mouse heart by oral application of tamoxifen citrate. Genesis, (2007) 45(1): 11–16. https://doi.org/10.1002/dvg.20244

13. Yoshinobu K, Araki M, Morita A, Araki M, Kokuba S, Nakagata N, Araki K (2021) Tamoxifen feeding method is suitable for efficient conditional knockout. Exp Anim 70(1): 91–100. https://doi.org/10.1538/expanim.19-0138

14. Smith BM, Saulsbery AI, Sarchet P, Devasthali N, Einstein D, Kirby ED (2022) Oral and injected tamoxifen alter adult hippocampal neurogenesis in female and male mice. eNeuro 9(2):ENEURO.0422-21.2022. https://doi.org/10.1523/eneuro.0422-21.2022

15. Harper MJK, Walpole AL (1967) A new derivative of triphenylethylene: effect on implantation and mode of action in rats. Reproduction 13(1):101–119. https://doi.org/10.1530/jrf.0.0130101

16. Madisen L, Zwingman TA, Sunkin SM, Oh SW, Zariwala HA, Gu H, Ng LL, Palmiter RD, Hawrylycz MJ, Jones AR, Lein ES, Zeng H (2010) A robust and high-throughput Cre reporting and characterization system for the whole mouse brain. Nat Neurosci 13(1): 133–140. https://doi.org/10.1038/nn.2467

17. Madisen L, Garner AR, Shimaoka D, Chuong AS, Klapoetke NC, Li L, van der Bourg A, Niino Y, Egolf L, Monetti C, Gu H, Mills M, Cheng A, Tasic B, Nguyen TN, Sunkin SM, Benucci A, Nagy A, Miyawaki A, Helmchen F, Empson RM, Knöpfel T, Boyden ES, Reid RC, Carandini M, Zeng H (2015) Transgenic mice for intersectional targeting of neural sensors and effectors with high specificity and performance. Neuron 85(5):942–958. https://doi.org/10.1016/j.neuron.2015.02.022

Chapter 15

Techniques in Staining of Rodent and Human Olfactory Tissue

Hironobu Nishijima and Eric H. Holbrook

Abstract

Staining of olfactory tissue allows for evaluation of the organization of specific cell types within the specimen and allows for assessment in abnormalities of function that may be related to changes in normal tissue architecture. Histochemical staining and immunohistochemical (IHC) techniques are the most common methods for visualizing olfactory epithelium and olfactory bulbs. Here we describe the method of IHC for olfactory tissue utilizing both fluorescent and peroxidase-based methods of visualization.

Key words Olfactory epithelium, Olfactory bulbs, Immunohistochemistry, Immunofluorescence

1 Introduction

Histology of the olfactory tissue has mostly been concentrated on the olfactory epithelium and olfactory bulb utilizing staining procedures to identify specific cells of the system or neuropathways and synaptic targets. Although transgenic animals expressing tags to identify cells expressing mRNA of proteins mostly unique to the cell type of interest are now commonly used, the majority of histologic analysis relies on immunohistochemistry for visualizing components of the olfactory system. Immunohistochemistry is a method to examine the localization of target proteins in tissues by reacting them with antibodies that specifically recognize antigen sites of unique proteins present in cells or the extracellular matrix. Conjugated antibodies are typically visualized by either enzyme-mediated staining or fluorescent tags.

In the study of olfaction, histological studies are often performed on olfactory mucosal tissue, but the olfactory bulbs are also common areas of investigation. This requires a detailed understanding of the anatomy of the human and animal (mainly rodent) nasal cavity with surrounding structures. The nasal cavity of the mouse, like that of humans, consists of the right and left nasal

Bradley J. Goldstein and Hiroaki Matsunami (eds.), *The Olfactory System*, Methods in Molecular Biology, vol. 2710,
https://doi.org/10.1007/978-1-0716-3425-7_15,

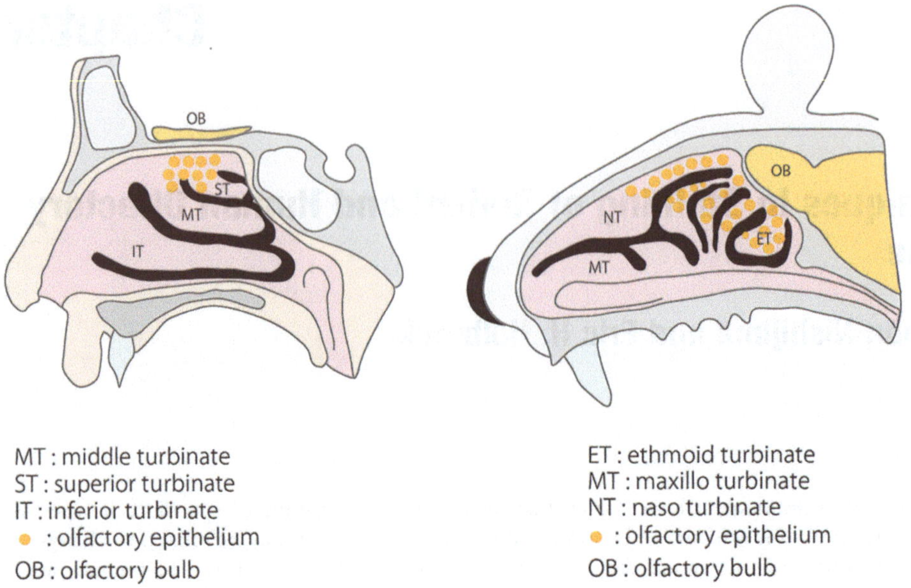

Fig. 1 Illustration of the lateral mucosa of the nasal cavity of human (left) and mouse (right). In humans, olfactory epithelium is present in the uppermost parts of the middle turbinate, superior turbinate and nasal septum [5]. In contrast, in mouse the olfactory epithelium is more extensive and present throughout the cribriform turbinate in the posterior half of the lateral wall and posterior-superior septum

passages, the nasal concha and the nasal septum (Fig. 1). Multiple nasal turbinates are present on the outer lateral wall of the nasal cavity. The human nasal cavity consists of the inferior, middle, and superior nasal turbinates, while the mouse nasal turbinates are largely divided into the anteriorly located nasoturbinate and maxilloturbinate, and posteriorly located ethmoid turbinate [1, 2]. In humans, olfactory neuroepithelium is restricted to a very limited area of medial surface of the middle and superior turbinate and uppermost part of the nasal septum, whereas most of the ethmoidal turbinates in mice contain olfactory neuroepithelium [1–6].

This paper describes general immunohistochemical staining as well as specific information pertinent to olfactory tissue staining. These basic guidelines refer mostly to common staining of tissue sections but can also be extrapolated for use in staining of epithelial sheets or whole tissue preparations or combined with other techniques such as tissue clearing procedures. Throughout this paper, the method for frozen sections will be designated as (Fr) and the method for paraffin sections as (Pa). Methods not specified for either are common for both section types. For immunostaining, the fluorescent staining methods are designated as (Fl) and the enzyme-antibody method as (En). Methods not specified for either are common to both labeling techniques. When provided in the methods, listed manufacturers were those commonly used for our staining. However, many manufacturers of antibody complexes and staining reagents are available for similar purposes, and we do not imply any advantage of one company over others.

2 Materials

Prepare and store all reagents at room temperature (unless indicated otherwise).

1. ***Animal model preparation***
   - (a) Anesthesia: ketamine 80–100 mg/kg + xylazine 5–10 mg/kg (intraperitoneal injection).
   - (b) Dissection tools: scissors, scalpel, forceps, rongeur.
2. ***Fixation***
   - (a) Instruments for perfusion fixation.
   - (b) Common fixatives include 10% neutral buffered formalin solution, or 4% paraformaldehyde solution (*see* **Note 1**).
3. ***Decalcification***
   - (a) Bottle or 50 ml Falcon tube.
   - (b) 10% EDTA.
4. ***Embedding***
   - (a) Embedding molds or containers made of aluminum foil, vacuum bell.

     (F): Sucrose gradient: 10%, 20%, 30%, 50 mL each (for rodent nasal tissue).

     Optimal Cutting Temperature (OCT) embedding media.

     (P): Paraffin.
5. ***Sectioning***
   - (a) Cryostat (F) or microtome (P).
   - (b) Protein coated, adhesive, or electrostatically charged microscope slides (Plus Slides, Thermo Fisher Scientific, Pittsburg, PA) provide enhanced section adherence.
6. ***Immunohistochemistry.***

2.6.1 Equipment

- (a) Staining (Coplin) jars, slide rack, hydrophobic blocking pen or rubber cement, and moist chamber.
- (b) Buffered base solution: phosphate-buffered saline (PBS, 10X stock solution): To 800 ml ddH_2O add 80 g NaCl, 2 g KCl, 27.2 g $Na_2HPO_4(H_2O)7$, and 2.4 g KH_2PO_4. Bring pH to 7.4, bring volume to 1 L in ddH_2O. This concentrated stock solution requires 1:10 dilution in water for use.

2.6.2. Antigen Retrieval

(a) Heat-induced epitope retrieval: can include autoclave, rice steamer, microwave oven, hot water heater, etc.

(b) 0.01 M citric acid buffer: 1.235 g sodium citrate dihydrate (MW 247 g/mol) for 500 ml adjust pH to 6.0 (*see* **Note 2**).

2.6.3. Protein Background Blocking (to Decrease Nonspecific Antibody Staining)

Block solution: 4% bovine serum albumin (BSA) in PBS with 5% Nonfat dry milk. Add 10% animal serum (*see* **Note 3**).

2.6.4. Blocking Endogenous Peroxidase Activity for Peroxidase Base Staining

3% hydrogen peroxide water in PBS (*see* **Note 4**).

7. ***Primary antigens and conjugates***

   (a) Table 1 provides a list of common antibodies used with immunohistochemistry for identifying epithelial cell types of the olfactory epithelium and bulb [5, 6].

   (b) Figure 3 provides representative images of olfactory epithelium and bulb labeled with several cell specific antibodies.

   (c) Primary antibody dilution in base blocking buffer: 1% BSA, 0.3% Triton x-100 in PBS.

8. ***Secondary antibody reagents***

   (a) Biotinylated secondary antibodies.

   (b) (En) Directly conjugated peroxidase secondary antibody or biotinylated secondary antibody with avidin-biotinylated horse radish peroxidase kits.

   (c) (Fl) Fluorescent streptavidin complexes or directly conjugated fluorescent labeled secondary antibody.

9. ***Light-based visualization***

   (En) Peroxidase-based staining often utilizes 3,3′-diaminobenzadine (DAB) as the chromogen. Other similar chromogens are available as a substitute for DAB.

10. ***Nuclear staining***

   (a) (Fl): Blue-emitting 4′,6-diamidino-2-phenylindole (DAPI) or Hoechst 33342 under UV wavelength.

   (b) (En): Hematoxylin is commonly used with enzyme-antibody methods visualized under light microscopy. Eosin is sometimes used to show extracellular matrix and cell membranes (*see* **Note 5**).

Table 1
Selected primary antibodies and cell type-sdpecific labeling

Primary antibody	Target cell
OMP	Mature OSNs
PGP 9.5	OSNs
TUBB3/TUJ1	OSNs
GAP43	Immature OSNs
SOX2	Upstream GBCs HBCs, sustentacular cells
SOX9	Bowman's gland and ducts
KI 67	Proliferating cells
CK5, CK14, p63	HBCs
TUBB4	RE sustentacular cells
CK19	RE sustentacular cells, HBCs
CK18	Sustentacular cells
VGlUT2	Glomerular synapses in OB

Abbreviations: *OSNs* olfactory sensory neurons, *GBCs* globose basal cells, *HBCs* horizontal basal cells, *RE* respiratory epithelium, *OMP* olfactory marker protein, *PGP 9.5* protein gene product 9.5, *TUBB3* Beta 3 tubulin, *GAP43* anti-growth-associated protein-43, *SOX2* SRY (sex determining region Y)-box 2, *SOX9* SRY (sex determining region Y)-box 9, *CK5* Cytokeratin5, *CK14* Cytokeratin14, *TUBB4* Beta 4 tubulin, *CK19* Cytokeratin19, *CK18* Cytokeratin18, *VGLuT2* vesicular glutamate transporter 2

11. ***Signal amplification***
    (a) (Fl) Tyramide signal amplification (TSA) is an example of a commonly used method we have used to enhance fluorescent signals, per manufacturer instructions (PerkinElmer, Waltham, MA).
    (b) (En) Methods include: Avidin-biotinylated peroxidase method (ABC method), labeled streptavidin biotinylated peroxidase method (LSAB method), Envision Method (Dako) using polymers with peroxidase (horseradish peroxidase: HRP) conjugated to secondary antibodies.
12. ***Slide mounting***
    (a) (Fl) Rinse with PBS. Coverslip with mounting medium, 0.1 M n-propyl gallate.
    (b) (En) Gradient ethanol, xylene required for most peroxidase and precipitate labeling methods. Coverslip with DPX nonaqueous mounting medium.

3 Methods

The following procedures are performed at room temperature unless otherwise specified.

1. ***Specimen acquisition***
   (a) With whole head specimens of rodents, intracardiac perfusion of fixative is performed at a slow rate after saline or PBS clearing of blood, the whole body is perfused or the aorta is clamped to provide the majority of fixative to the head. The head is removed, and excessive surrounding soft tissue and bone are carefully dissected away using rongeurs and dissecting scissors from the nasal cavity (e.g., mandible bone).
   (b) Specimens obtained from human surgical cases or clinic biopsies can be immediately immersed in fixative. Orientation of specimen should be preserved if possible (*see* **Note 6**).
2. ***Specimen preparation***
   (a) Specimens are further immersed in fixative solution at room temperature for several hours to several days. Specimens are then immersed in a decalcification solution for several days to a week depending on bone thickness until the remaining bone is soft (*see* **Note 7**).
   (b) The decalcified head is embedded in OTC or paraffin for block preparation taking care to maintain orientation (*see* **Note 8**). In preparation for obtaining frozen sections, soak the specimens and submerge sequentially in a series of 10%, 20%, and 30% sucrose solutions at 4 °C until the specimens sink at each concentration. We typically utilize liquid nitrogen for flash freezing of tissue within OCT (*see* **Note 9**).
   (c) The tissue block is routinely positioned in the microtome or cryostat for obtaining sections in the coronal plane (*see* **Note 10**).
   (d) With human biopsy tissue, every attempt should be made to orient the specimens so that sections are obtained through a perpendicular plane to the epithelial surface (*see* **Note 11**).
   (e) Sections should be 10–20 μm thick for frozen sections and 4 μm thick for paraffin sections depending on the need for visualization of various cells or structures and mounted on glass slides.

3. ***Immunohistochemistry***

   3.3.1. cleaning and hydration of sections

   (a) (Fr) For frozen sections, soak in PBS to remove the embedding agent 3–5 min.

   (b) (Pa) For paraffin sections, deparaffinize and hydrate by soaking in xylene followed by decreasing concentrations of ethanol (100 to 70%) and PBS.

4. ***Antigen retrieval***

   (a) Steam method: this method is most common in our use. Create a water-repellent circle around the specimen area with a PAP hydrophobic pen. Pour the citrate reagent over the specimen well. Heat the specimen in the steamer at 45 °C for 10 min. Be careful not to allow the specimen to dry out.

   (b) Autoclave method: place the citrate reagent on glass slides in a heat-resistant container with a lid. Heat in an autoclave at 120 °C for 10 min.

   (c) After cooling, wash sections with PBS.

5. ***Inactivation of endogenous enzymes***

   Immerse slides in 3% (v/v) hydrogen peroxide. Reaction time is usually 5 to 20 min; rinse with PBS (*see* **Note 12**).

6. ***Blocking nonspecific protein interaction***

   Place the blocking solution on the sections and allow to stand at room temperature for about 1 h (*see* **Note 13**).

7. ***Primary antibody conjugation***

   Carefully remove block solution from sections, apply the primary antibody solution to the sections, and incubate at room temperature for 1 h or at 4 °C overnight (*see* **Note 14**).

8. ***Secondary antibody conjugation***

   After primary antibody incubation, thoroughly wash tissue with buffer solution (PBS wash). If the primary antibody is labeled with an enzyme, perform the enzyme reaction for visualization (direct method). If the primary antibody is unlabeled, add the appropriate secondary antibody to identify the Fc portion of the primary antibody (indirect method). The secondary antibody is reacted at room temperature for approximately 1 h at the manufacturer specified concentration (*see* **Note 15**).

   (Fl) In our practice, primary antibodies are visualized either by incubating with the corresponding biotinylated secondary antibody (Jackson ImmunoResearch Laboratories, Inc., West Grove, PA) followed by fluorescent streptavidin complexes (tertiary reagent) to strengthen the signal or with a suitable fluorescent tagged secondary antibody (Invitrogen, ThermoFisher Scientific, Waltham, MA).

(En) Primary antibodies are visualized either by incubating with the corresponding biotinylated secondary antibody (Jackson ImmunoResearch Laboratories, Inc., West Grove, PA) followed by biotinylated horseradish peroxidase (bHRP) activated with chromagen solution to increase signal or with a peroxidase conjugated secondary antibody followed by chromagen activation. Staining is most often visualized using 3,3′-diaminobenzadine (DAB) as the chromogen.

9. ***Signal amplification***

Several commercially available signal amplification kits are available to increase the intensity of antibody staining which is beyond the scope of this paper. It is important to realize when signal enhancement is used, nonspecific binding is also enhanced; it is advisable to stain an appropriate negative control at the same time.

10. ***Nuclear staining to identify all cells of the tissue for contrast with specific antigen staining***
    (a) (Fl) Apply DAPI or Hoechst 33342 to the slides for 10 min. If nuclear signal is too light, make fresh solution or lengthen application. Rinse with PBS.
    (b) (En) Wash glass slides with distilled water. Immerse slides in hematoxylin solution for 30 s to 2 min. Rinse under gentle running water to avoid overstaining.

11. ***Coverslip mounting***
    (a) (Fl) Coverslip slides with 0.1 M n-propyl gallate to decrease bleaching of signal. Drain excess mounting media to prevent uneven thickness. The coverslip can be sealed with fingernail polish to prevent loss of mounting media over time. Store at a cold temperature or freeze slides in the dark. Avoid freeze-thaw cycles.
    (b) (En) Dehydrate stained slides through increasing concentrations of ethanol up to 100% and clear with xylene. Coverslip with DPX mounting media.

4 Notes

1. Both fixative solutions will work for optical microscopy. 4% PFA should be prepared fresh when needed. Numerous fixatives have been described, and variations may be required

depending on needs and sensitivity of specific antigens of interest.

2. Heat sections in 0.01 M citrate buffer, pH 6.0, but if antigen activation is insufficient, try pH 7 and pH 8, or other solutions with surfactants. Antigen activation re-exposes target antigens on the surface that have been denatured in formalin-fixed specimens or during preparation. We commonly use heat-related antigen retrieval methods; however other published techniques such as proteolytic enzymes, for example, are available.
3. We typically use serum from the same species as the secondary antibodies used in staining. Commercialized blocking solutions are also available.
4. Hydrogen peroxide should be diluted just before application to prevent diminishing effect from prolonged time and exposure to light. When endogenous peroxidase activity is high (especially in frozen sections), the oxygen generated by the reaction with hydrogen peroxide may form bubbles and cause tissue damage or peeling. In such cases, methanol is used as a diluent. However, for certain cell surface antigens, the combination of methanol and hydrogen peroxide may cause denaturation of the epitope resulting in a failure of the antibody reaction.
5. It is recommended that nuclear staining be performed to clarify the localization of all cells within the tissue of interest. In fluorescence staining, nuclear staining is also helpful for determining cell depth and for use as a focusing target.
6. When obtaining human olfactory epithelium specimens from living subjects, the location of the biopsy is critically important. If the biopsy is obtained under general anesthesia, the superior turbinate can be a good source of olfactory epithelium. The anterior olfactory epithelium on the septum can be accessed with minimal discomfort for small biopsies in awake patients. In either case, delicate handling of the specimen is required as epithelial denudement can easily occur. Please see Holbrook, et al. (2016) for more detailed description of biopsies for human olfactory epithelium [3].
7. Allow the EDTA to decalcify the bone until it is soft and can be cut with a knife. The amount of EDTA should be about 20 times that of the specimen, and the EDTA solution should be changed during the decalcification process. Remove any hard bone (skull, palate, etc.) that is not necessary for analysis before demineralization to speed up the process. Incomplete decalcification can result in poor histologic sections and defects through the tissue from dragging fragments at the blade edge.
8. The classification of Young et al. is often used to classify the levels of the coronal section of the nasal cavity in rodents [7]. It

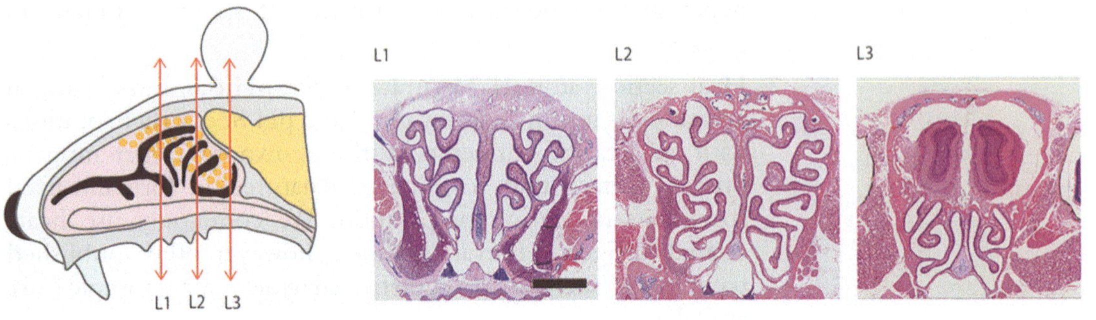

Fig. 2 Coronal paraffin sections of mouse nasal cavity stained with hematoxylin and eosin. In L1, the lower half is respiratory epithelium, and the upper half is olfactory epithelium. In L2, most of the nasal cavity is covered with olfactory epithelium. In L3, the upper half contains the olfactory bulbs, and the lower half contains the posterior nasal cavity with mix of olfactory and respiratory epithelium. Scale bar: 1 mm

is described as four spaced sections in the coronal plane: level 1 is immediately posterior to the upper incisor teeth, level 2 is at the incisive papilla, level 3 is at the second palatal ridge, and level 4 is at the level of the first upper molar teeth. Level 1 is suitable for evaluation of the respiratory mucosa. Level 2 is used to evaluate the anterior part of the olfactory mucosa, level 3 is used to evaluate the center of the olfactory mucosa, and level 4 is used to evaluate the posterior part of the olfactory mucosa and the olfactory bulb. Figure 2 shows a section of the coronal section just anterior to the anterior end of the olfactory bulb, which is visible through the parietal bone, and used as a landmark (Young level 3). This cross section is approximately the same as the most anterior end of eye. This cross section is commonly sampled because the sampling of the ethmoidal turbinates is greatest.

9. Tissue damage due to ice crystal formation during freezing affects the histological image of frozen sections. The damage can be minimized by using sucrose. In addition, over freezing the tissue block can result in fracturing of the tissue block. Removal of tissue from liquid nitrogen just before complete freezing and placement on dry ice or in −80 ° C freezer can reduce fracturing. In addition, limiting total OCT surrounding the tissue by creating smaller molds can reduce fracturing.
10. During fixative solution penetration and embedding, a vacuum should be used to remove air contained in the space between the nasal turbinate to ensure that the solution is distributed evenly to all areas.
11. Tissue sections through the epithelium tangential to the basal lamina and not in the perpendicular plane will give the appearance of thicker epithelium, distort the morphology of component cells, and may falsely demonstrate multiple layers of specific cell types (e.g., horizontal basal cell layer).

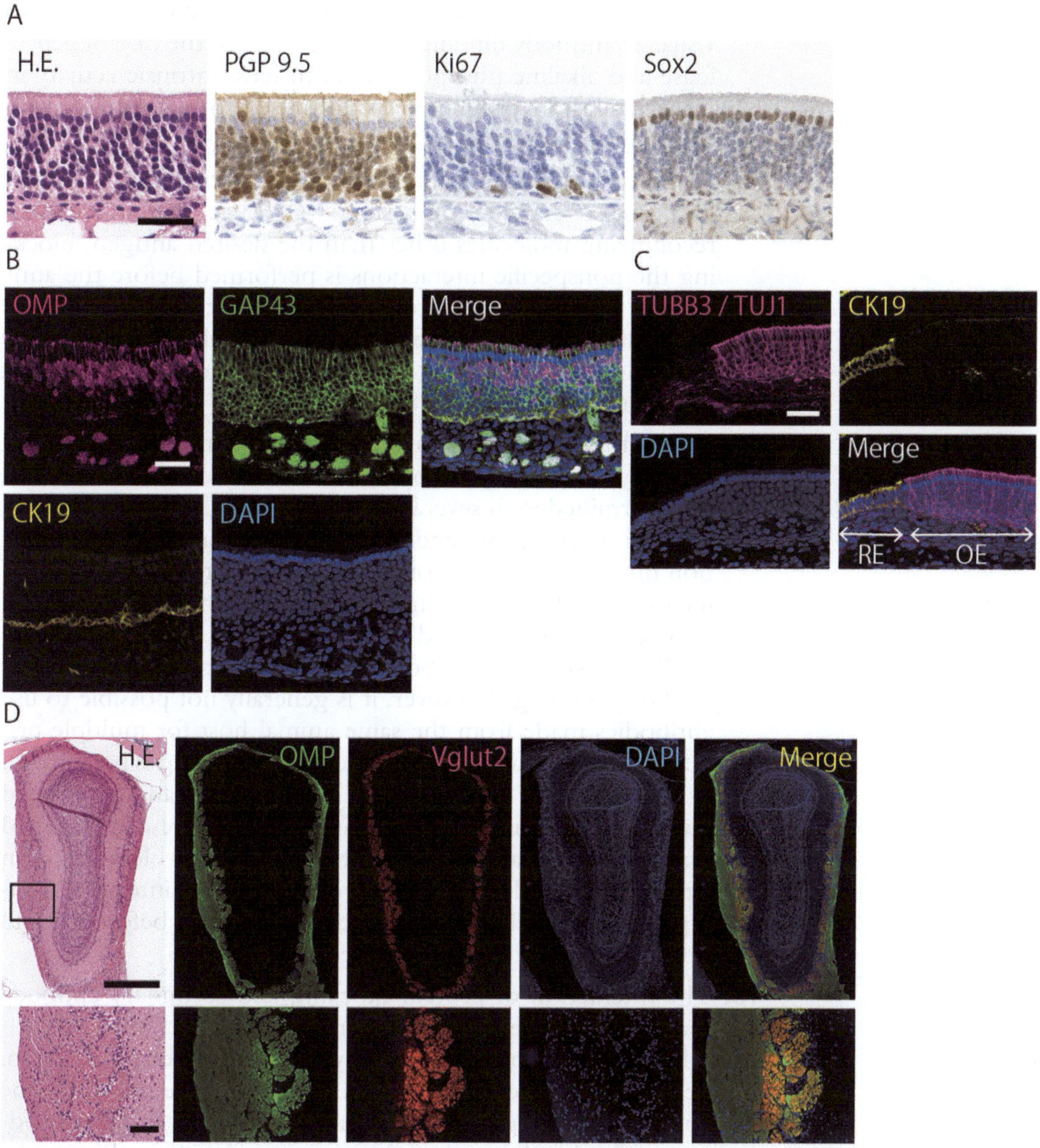

Fig. 3 (**a**) Examples of paraffin sections through mouse olfactory epithelium stained with hematoxylin and eosin (HE) and followed by antibody staining to various common antibodies visualized with enzyme-peroxidase method and DAB as a chromagen. The antibody-stained sections were counterstained with hematoxylin. Scale bar: 25 μm. (**b**) Examples of frozen sections through mouse olfactory epithelium stained with various common antibodies and viewed with fluorescence. Scale bar: 25 μm. (**c**) The boundary between olfactory epithelium and respiratory epithelium can be better delineated with immunohistochemistry. Frozen sections of mouse nasal mucosa labeled with epithelium specific antibodies and fluorescent markers. RE, respiratory epithelium; OE, olfactory epithelium; scale bar, 25 μm. (**d**) Coronal paraffin sections through the right mouse olfactory bulb. HE staining (left image) is followed by examples of antibody labeling with fluorescent markers. Scale bar: 500 μm. The lower row provides a higher magnification of the area indicated by the box in the upper row and highlights the glomeruli. Scale bar: 50 μm

12. Necessity for this step depends on which enzyme is used to visualize antibody binding to the antigen. In the case of peroxidase and alkaline phosphatase, both have intrinsic activity in many tissues. Hydrogen peroxide is used to inactivate peroxidase, but this inactivation is irreversible.
13. Nonspecific binding of antibodies is a factor that increases background staining of tissue. To reduce antibodies from recognizing molecules other than the desired antigen, blocking the nonspecific interactions is performed before the antibody is applied. In addition, during the reaction with primary antibodies, simple blocking with BSA can also be performed. When using animal serum for blocking, do not use same serum source as the primary antibody species.
14. Dilute the antibody with buffered solution such as PBS or blocking solution. The optimal antibody concentration can be determined with several dilutions using the antibody product data sheet recommendation as a starting reference. Incubation duration beyond room temperature for 1 h or overnight incubation (4 °C) can enhance signal strength but must be weighed against increased background.

    The fluorescent antibody method allows for easy multiple antibody staining. However, it is generally not possible to use antibodies made from the same animal host for multiple primary antibody staining unless sequential staining is performed.

    Be aware of the effects of natural light and prolonged fluorescent microscope exposure on fluorescent tagged reagents and stained tissue sections. Photo-bleaching can occur rapidly and diminish or even remove the intended staining. Antibodies should be diluted immediately before use and not repeatedly frozen and thawed.
15. The interaction of protein blocking and secondary antibody may produce unexpected background. To check the compatibility of the secondary antibody with the blocking solution, perform the procedure without the primary antibody. If the background is high, try increasing the dilution of the secondary antibody, shortening the reaction time, or change the blocking agent.

References

1. Harkema JR (1991) Comparative aspects of nasal airway anatomy: relevance to inhalation toxicology. Toxicol Pathol 19:321–336
2. Mery S, Gross EA, Joyner DR, Godo M, Morgan KT (1994) Nasal diagrams: a tool for recording the distribution of nasal lesions in rats and mice. Toxicol Pathol 22:353–372
3. Holbrook EH, Rebeiz L, Schwob JE (2016) Office-based olfactory mucosa biopsies. Int Forum of Allergy Rhinol 6:646–653
4. Nishijima H, Zunitch MJ, Yoshida M, Kondo K, Yamasoba T, Schwob JE, Holbrook EH (2022) Rapid fluorescent vital imaging of olfactory epithelium. iScience 25:104222

5. Fitzek M, Patel PK, Solomon PD, Lin B, Hummel T, Schwob JE, Holbrook EH (2022) Integrated age-related immunohistological changes occur in human olfactory epithelium and olfactory bulb. J Comp Neurol 530:2154–2175
6. Child KM, Herrick DB, Schwob JE, Holbrook EH, Jang W (2018) The neuroregenerative capacity of olfactory stem cells is not limitless: implications for aging. J Neurosci 38:6806–6824
7. Young JT (1981) Histopathologic examination of the rat nasal cavity. Fundam Appl Toxicol 1: 309–312

[illegible]

Chapter 16

Electrophysiological Recordings from Identified Cell Types in the Olfactory Cortex of Awake Mice

Kevin A. Bolding and Kevin M. Franks

Abstract

Neural circuits consist of a myriad of distinct cell types, each with specific intrinsic properties and patterns of synaptic connectivity, which transform neural input and convey this information to downstream targets. Understanding how different features of an odor stimulus are encoded and relayed to their appropriate targets will require selective identification and manipulation of these different elements of the circuit. Here, we describe methods to obtain dense, extracellular electrophysiological recordings of odor-evoked activity in olfactory (piriform) cortex of awake, head-fixed mice, and optogenetic tools and procedures to identify genetically defined cell types within this circuit.

Key words Piriform cortex, In vivo electrophysiology, Cell types, Optogenetics

1 Introduction

Electrophysiological methods for monitoring the activity of individual neurons during sensory stimulation or behavior have provided fundamental insights into how features of the external world are reflected in neural activity. Foundational work recording from one or a few neurons allowed localization of sensory or motor functions to specific brain regions [1–6]. The description of differing single neuron responses or "tuning" as stimuli or behavioral output programs are progressively processed by connected brain regions has inspired our field's fundamental models for neural computation and brain function.

However, many individual neurons do not display clear and obvious tuning properties [7, 8]. Moreover, downstream areas rarely receive input from single neurons. Analyses of neural activity at the population level is therefore essential for understanding what neurons are encoding and how they are affecting downstream areas [9, 10]. The recent transformative development in multielectrode recording now allows us to ask how populations of neurons,

Bradley J. Goldstein and Hiroaki Matsunami (eds.), *The Olfactory System*, Methods in Molecular Biology, vol. 2710,
https://doi.org/10.1007/978-1-0716-3425-7_16,

working in concert, can efficiently encode information and carry out computations [11, 12]. Interactions between distinct neural populations within and across brain regions shape neural activity to enable perception and behavior [13–16]. Principal neurons within a region share physiological properties and receive inputs with similar information content and statistical properties, leading to a degree of functional specialization within each region [17, 18]. We can gain insight into the specific way that different regions transform information by contrasting activity in neural populations in connected regions. To this end, we and others have recorded from multiple regions of the mouse olfactory system responding to the same stimuli [19–24]. By recording simultaneously from different regions in the same animal, we can ensure that changes in neural responses between regions are not explained by differences across animals or across recording sessions. This approach further presents the opportunity to investigate the nature and dynamics of information transfer between regions [21, 22].

Neural circuits are composed of distinct cell types that perform different specific functions to transform neural information [25–30]. Prior to the development and widespread adoption of optogenetic methods, cell types could only be identified in extracellular electrophysiological recordings by their characteristic spike waveforms, recording location, and other features of their spiking activity (e.g., rhythmicity, bursting) [31–36]. The combination of optogenetic actuators to increase or decrease a neuron's activity [37–41], the refinement of conditional viral vectors to robustly express these optogenetic tools in defined cell types [42, 43], and a growing library of "driver" mouse lines that confer molecular specificity for where these proteins are expressed have made it possible to label cells according to their lineage, connectivity, or even their activity during defined experimental epochs [44, 45]. During in vivo recordings, optogenetic stimulation is used to drive or inhibit the targeted cells' activity and "tag" them, so that cells of a given type can be identified in subsequent analyses. Opto-tagging thus allows us to determine the interactions between cell types in a region and how they shape computation within a neural circuit.

Here we describe methods for multi-region recording with extracellular multielectrode arrays and opto-tagging to identify inhibitory and excitatory cell types in the main olfactory system [20–22, 46]. The basic framework we provide here is adaptable for investigating neural coding and computation in almost any brain area.

2 Materials and Methods

1. *Prepare rig and materials for head-fixed electrophysiological recording.*
   1.1. The primary requirements for a headpost design are that the headpost material does not produce an inflammatory response, the craniotomy site required to target the region of interest is accessible, and the materials are inflexible enough to prevent head movement [47, 48]. Designs using 3D printed plastic or steel, laser-cut titanium or steel, or CNC-machined parts have been successfully used in this application. Numerous open-source designs are available (Table 1).
   1.2. Manual or computer-controlled micromanipulators are used to precisely position the electrode in the target region (*see* **Note 1**).
   1.3. Make ground and reference pins. We constructed pins by inserting a short piece of 0.008″ bare silver wire (A-M systems, #786500 or #782000) into the base of a male connector pin (A-M systems, #520100) and allowing melted solder to run into the internal cavity of the pins to create a contact and fix the wire in place. These are trimmed so that the wire extends from the base of the pin by ~1 mm.
2. *Cell type-specific expression of excitatory or inhibitory opsins.*
   2.1. Transgenic mouse lines are available from commercial vendors that express excitatory or inhibitory opsins in specific cell types. Transgenic lines have the advantage that no further preparation is required to enable optogenetic tagging experiments. The primary disadvantage of this approach is that genetic manipulations and long-term expression of opsins may affect physiology or behavior (*see* **Note 2**).
   2.2. Numerous strategies combine transgenic methods with viral opsin expression or virus delivery alone to produce

Table 1
Example headpost design resources

Reference	Link
Huber et al., 2012 [49]	Janelia Research Campus - Open Science
Osborne and Dudman, 2014 [50]	Dudman Lab – RIVETS
The International Brain Laboratory et al., 2021 [51]	IBL protocol for headbar implant surgery in mice

optogenetic control with spatiotemporally restricted and cell type-specific opsin expression.

2.3. Detailed protocols for stereotaxic delivery of viral vectors are available [38, 52]. Our strategy for expressing inhibitory opsins in a Cre recombinase expressing cell type in piriform cortex is described briefly here:

(a) Animals are anesthetized and placed in a stereotaxic frame and maintained on isoflurane anesthesia (0.5–2% in 0.8 L/min O_2) throughout the procedure.

(b) A local anesthetic, bupivacaine, is injected under the skin over the skull, and an incision is made along the midline to expose the skull.

(c) Between one and four burr holes, depending on the experiment, are made at the injection target coordinates.

(d) AAVs (either AAV8-hSyn-DIO-Jaws-eYFP or AAV5-hSyn-DIO-ArchT3.0-eYFP, obtained from UNC Vector Core), are then delivered through a glass pipette using a Nanoject pump (Drummond) (200 nL/site at 60 nL/min).

(e) After slowly retracting the pipette, burr holes are covered using Kwik-Cast sealant.

(f) Viral injection surgery can be combined with headpost implantation. After 3–4 weeks to allow viral expression, a second brief surgery will be required to make a craniotomy for probe placement at the recording site.

3. *Implant a headpost and ground/reference pins.*

3.1. Anesthetize and prepare the animal for surgery, and place the animal in the stereotaxic apparatus.

3.2. In preparing the animal for headpost implantation, it is critical to achieve a clean and dry skull surface to which dental cement can adhere effectively. This requires scraping the skull with a scalpel blade or specialized scraping tool to remove the periosteum, paying special attention to the skull sutures. Further, the skull should be cleaned with sterile saline until no blood is present at any cement attachment. Remaining periosteum or blood can cause inflammation and compromise head fixation and tissue health.

3.3. Using an FG ¼ or smaller dental drill bit, drill two small burr holes over the cerebellum with 3–4 mm spacing between holes to allow contact of ground and reference pins with brain surface/cerebrospinal fluid.

3.4. Attach a syringe needle or pipette to the stereotaxic arm and level the skull by adjusting the bite bar position until the Z coordinates of bregma and lambda are within 20 microns of each other. It is useful to keep additional records of the Z coordinates at locations 2–3 mm lateral to these landmarks on either side to identify systematic errors and quantify the variance in roll axis for stereotaxis positioning.

3.5. Identify the appropriate probe insertion site(s) by stereotaxic coordinates and drill a small (1–2 mm diameter) craniotomy for each.

3.6. It will be necessary to clean the skull again to remove bone dust and blood from these drilling operations before applying any adhesives.

3.7. Cover the probe craniotomy with a small plug of Kwik-Cast. This Kwik-Cast can be mixed together in a small amount and applied while still runny using a bent syringe needle.

3.8. To implant ground and reference pins, use a syringe needle to apply a small amount of Krazy glue to the base, making sure to leave the wire exposed, and use forceps to hold the pin and position the wire in the burr hole over the cerebellum. Krazy glue will hold the pins in place until the application of dental cement to fix the headpost and pins in place (*see* **Note 3**).

3.9. Attach the headpost to a stereotaxic arm. We have achieved this by replacing the stereotaxic arm with a machined post with a threaded end (available from commercial optics companies) and inserting a cap screw through the headpost hole used for the headpost holder. Solutions to this task vary by headpost type but usually take the form of imitating the rig's headpost holder design on a stereotaxic arm.

3.10. Position the headpost so that it is just touching the skull. The craniotomy should be accessible with the headpost in place. It is important to consider the width and depth of your recording probe when determining accessibility.

3.11. Apply dental cement to fix the headpost and ground and reference pins to the skull.

3.12. Release the headpost from the stereotaxic arm, and wait for dental cement to solidify.

3.13. Proceed with standard postoperative recovery protocol. Recordings should be made as soon as possible in accordance with institutional animal care guidelines to ensure integrity of the craniotomy over the recording site.

4. *Acute electrophysiological recording and optogenetic tagging in head-fixed animals*

   4.1. After opsin expression has been achieved and the animal has recovered from headpost and craniotomy surgeries, large-scale recording from identified cell populations can proceed.

   4.2. Electrophysiology system and probes: In our recordings, electrophysiological signals were acquired with a 32-site polytrode acute probe (A1-32-Poly3-5 mm-25 s-177, Neuronexus, Ann Arbor, MI) through an A32-OM32 adaptor (Neuronexus) connected to a Cereplex digital headstage (Blackrock Microsystems, Salt Lake City, UT). Unfiltered signals were digitized at 30 kHz at the headstage and recorded by a Cerebus multichannel data acquisition system (BlackRock Microsystems). Many commercially available systems have similar acquisition capabilities. This approach is not dependent on the specific acquisition system. Experimental events and respiration signal were acquired at 2 kHz by analog inputs of the Cerebus system. Respiration was monitored with a microbridge mass airflow sensor (Honeywell AWM3300V, Morris Plains, NJ) positioned directly opposite the animal's nose. Prior to recording, the back of the probe can be painted with a fluorescent dye (diI, Life Technologies) to confirm probe positioning post hoc in histological sections.

   4.3. Optic fibers: We have used two configurations for optogenetic tagging. First, probes can be obtained from commercial vendors that have an optic fiber attached with glue, so that light is guaranteed to be distributed over the recorded tissue (e.g., A1-32-Poly3-5 mm-25 s-177-OA32LP, Neuronexus). Second, we have positioned 200 μm or 400 μm optic fibers at an angle using a separate micromanipulator to target light distribution to the recorded tissue. In either case, the optic fiber is coupled to a laser light source (Opto Engine LLC) of the appropriate wavelength using a patch cable (*see* **Note 4**).

   4.4. On the day of recording, lightly anesthetize the mouse with isoflurane (1% in O_2), drill away the cement over the craniotomy site, remove the Kwik-Cast, and remove the dura mater over the targeted insertion site for the recording probe:

(a). For recordings in anterior piriform cortex, position probe for insertion at 1.32 mm anterior and 3.8 mm lateral from bregma. Recordings should be targeted 3.5–4 mm ventral from the brain surface at this position with adjustment according to the local field potential (LFP) and spiking activity monitored online (*see* **Note 5**).

(b). For recordings in olfactory bulb, the probe can be positioned using coarse anatomical markings. The caudal boundary of the dorsal olfactory bulb is demarcated by the rostral rhinal vein, which is visible through the skull. The probe can be inserted anywhere near the center of the olfactory bulb, 1–2 mm lateral to the midline and 2–3 mm anterior to the rostral rhinal vein (*see* **Note 6**).

4.5. Laser pulses can be controlled via digital signals to switch the light source on or off or by inserting a mechanical shutter into the light path. The use of a shutter provides more precise control over the onset timing of light pulses, which is useful for latency-based optogenetic identification (*see* **Note 7**).

4.6. Opto-tagged cells can be identified by the change in their firing rate during laser stimulation and the latency of their change in firing after the onset of laser stimulation. A wide range of optogenetic tagging protocols has been applied successfully (*see* **Note 8**). We have previously used a protocol of 1000 pulses with a pulse duration of 300 ms to balance the requirements for pulse number and duration. Many fewer pulses can suffice when using an excitatory opsin for opto-tagging.

5. *Electrophysiology data processing and spike-sorting*

Because the specific steps for neural data processing are unique to each user's data and preferences for analysis pipeline, we will outline the steps at a high level and refer the reader to resources and tools that we have used in our research.

5.1. Obtain raw wideband electrophysiological data for the full set of data to be analyzed together. If separate recording files exist for the same session, they should be concatenated and processed together.

5.2. If data contains motion artifacts or other large voltage fluctuations that are outside of the high-frequency band of spiking activity, an internal reference signal can be subtracted from the data for electrode channels on the same recording probe to produce more reliable spike waveforms. Data should be high-pass filtered prior to referencing. The subtracted signal can come from a "quiet" channel with little spiking activity or an average of many channels (i.e., common average referencing). The averaged referencing procedure may be modified to adaptively select a subset of channels at each sample that are least likely to contain spiking activity.

5.3. Detect and assign spikes to extracellular units by clustering similar waveforms (i.e., spike-sorting). Recordings with dense multielectrode arrays require an automatic clustering step to assign spikes to specific units. Recent advances in clustering algorithms for neural data have improved both the speed and accuracy of this step. Many clustering algorithms are available as open-source packages (e.g., spyking-circus [53] and Kilosort [12, 54]; see also SpikeInterface [55]). Different packages implement varying degrees of pre-processing, including noise removal, detection of bad electrode channels, and high-pass filtering.

5.4. Clusters should be manually curated to remove units that have clearly artifactual waveforms or contain many spikes in the 1–2 ms refractory period revealed by constructing and visualizing each unit's auto-correlogram. When it's possible to identify "over-clustering" clusters may be merged (*see* **Note 9**).

6. *Classifying opto-tagged cells*

6.1. Excitatory opsins: Applying multiple criteria can increase confidence in true-positive identification for cells expressing ChR2 or other excitatory opsins. Relying on firing rate changes alone may produce many false positives due to network effects of optogenetic responses from other neurons:

(a) The stimulus-associated spike latency test (SALT) [56] provides a significance test for the change in spike latency distributions induced by light stimulation compared to a baseline period.

(b) We further require that the average response described by the PSTH of each unit relative to light pulse onset has a latency-to-peak response of <3 ms.

(c) With light pulses of greater length, a comparison can also be made between the spike counts during light pulses and the equivalent time period preceding stimulation. We have previously applied Wilcoxon rank-sum test to report the probability these firing rate changes occur by chance.

6.2. Inhibitory opsins: When using inhibitory opsins, stimulus-associated spike latency tests are no longer applicable. However, we can continue to use criteria related to the timing of activity suppression to improve confidence in optogenetic identification (*see* **Note 10**).

(a) We again use a Wilcoxon rank-sum test to assess firing rate changes between long-duration light pulses and the pre-stimulation period.

(b) Suppression should be rapid, so we further require that the median last-spike latency across all pulses is <10 ms.

(c) With a sufficient number of light pulses, it is possible to estimate the timing of the firing rate change induced stimulation using change point analysis [57, 58]. To do so, PSTHs are generated for each unit using 2 ms bins spanning 100 ms before to 100 ms after laser onset, and a change point within that time is determined using MATLAB's "find-changepts" function.

3 Notes

1. The micromanipulators should be mounted to the same surface as the headpost holders to assure precise alignment of the axis of electrode movement (i.e., approach angle) with the coordinate system of the animal's skull. The approach angle should be adjustable relative to the dorsal-ventral axis, and there must be a reliable relationship between user input and movement along the approach angle.
2. These animals should be compared to wild-type controls and carefully monitored for developmental abnormalities.
3. The previous drilling steps are likely to introduce movement in the stereotaxic coordinate location of the skull. It is recommended to re-level bregma and lambda just prior to attachment of the headpost.
4. When using a separate optic fiber, it is advisable to position the fiber before the recording probe to avoid disturbing the recorded tissue after the target recording location has been reached.
5. Electrode sites on the polytrode span 275 μm along the dorsal-ventral axis. Lower the probe until a band of intense spiking activity covering 30–40% of electrode sites near the correct ventral coordinate is observed. This activity reflects the densely packed layer II of piriform cortex. Under light anesthesia, LFP signals across all electrode sites in piriform cortex often show some synchronization with respiration.

6. To accommodate positioning of probes in olfactory bulb and ipsilateral piriform cortex, the olfactory bulb probe can be inserted at a 10-degree angle in the coronal plane. The probe should be lowered along this angle through the dorsal mitral cell and granule layers until encountering a dense band of high-frequency activity signifying the targeted ventrolateral mitral cell layer, typically between 1.2 and 1.8 mm from the bulb surface.
7. Optogenetic tagging: When recording stability is a concern, it may be advisable to bookend the entire recording session with laser stimulation pulses to increase confidence that an identified unit shows the same optogenetic response signature throughout the recording. Otherwise, stimulation should occur after all other important experimental events to avoid nonspecific perturbation of the neural population.
8. A longer stimulation time provides a better estimate of the firing rate, and a larger number of pulses improve confidence in response latency measures.
9. A unit's spikes may be separated due to drift in the recording probe's location in the tissue. Some clustering algorithms now take advantage of the density of electrode channels to track this drift and correct for it over time.
   - 9.1. In areas where neurons are known to spike in bursts, it is possible that a decrease in extracellular potential over the course of a burst will cause the unit to be separated into multiple clusters. These can be identified by the clear similarity of their scaled waveforms across multiple channels and a characteristic peak in the cross-correlogram of the clusters.
   - 9.2. A unit's spikes may also be separated into different clusters because of differences in its waveform during optogenetic drive. Optogenetic stimulation does not commonly make large changes in the extracellular waveform, but it is useful to attend to units that appear to exist only during or outside of the period of optogenetic stimulation.
10. Finally, because all inhibitory opto-tagging depends on a reduction in firing rate, cells with very low firing rates should be excluded from the dataset to avoid false negatives.

Acknowledgments

This work was supported by NIH grants DC009839, DC015525, DC016782, and U19 NS112953 and by Start-up funds from Duke University.

References

1. Hubel DH, Wiesel TN (1959) Receptive fields of single neurones in the cat's striate cortex. J Physiol 148:574–591
2. Hubel DH, Wiesel TN (1962) Receptive fields, binocular interaction and functional architecture in the cat's visual cortex. J Physiol 160(106–154):2
3. O'Keefe J, Dostrovsky J (1971) The hippocampus as a spatial map. Preliminary evidence from unit activity in the freely-moving rat. Brain Res 34:171–175. https://doi.org/10.1016/0006-8993(71)90358-1
4. O'Keefe J (1976) Place units in the hippocampus of the freely moving rat. Exp Neurol 51: 78–109. https://doi.org/10.1016/0014-4886(76)90055-8
5. Georgopoulos AP, Kalaska JF, Caminiti R, Massey JT (1982) On the relations between the direction of two-dimensional arm movements and cell discharge in primate motor cortex. J Neurosci 2:1527–1537. https://doi.org/10.1523/JNEUROSCI.02-11-01527.1982
6. Georgopoulos AP, Schwartz AB, Kettner RE (1986) Neuronal population coding of movement direction. Science 233:1416–1419. https://doi.org/10.1126/science.3749885
7. Rigotti M, Barak O, Warden MR et al (2013) The importance of mixed selectivity in complex cognitive tasks. Nature 497:585–590. https://doi.org/10.1038/nature12160
8. Kaufman MT, Benna MK, Rigotti M et al (2022) The implications of categorical and category-free mixed selectivity on representational geometries. Curr Opin Neurobiol 77: 102644. https://doi.org/10.1016/j.conb.2022.102644
9. Quian Quiroga R, Panzeri S (2009) Extracting information from neuronal populations: information theory and decoding approaches. Nat Rev Neurosci 10:173–185. https://doi.org/10.1038/nrn2578
10. Buzsáki G (2010) Neural syntax: cell assemblies, synapsembles and readers. Neuron 68: 362–385. https://doi.org/10.1016/j.neuron.2010.09.023
11. Buzsáki G (2004) Large-scale recording of neuronal ensembles. Nat Neurosci 7:446–451. https://doi.org/10.1038/nn1233
12. Steinmetz NA, Aydin C, Lebedeva A et al (2021) Neuropixels 2.0: a miniaturized high-density probe for stable, long-term brain recordings. Science 372:eabf4588. https://doi.org/10.1126/science.abf4588
13. Guo ZV, Li N, Huber D et al (2014) Flow of cortical activity underlying a tactile decision in mice. Neuron 81:179–194. https://doi.org/10.1016/j.neuron.2013.10.020
14. Semedo JD, Zandvakili A, Machens CK et al (2019) Cortical areas interact through a communication subspace. Neuron 102:249–259.e4. https://doi.org/10.1016/j.neuron.2019.01.026
15. Steinmetz NA, Zatka-Haas P, Carandini M, Harris KD (2019) Distributed coding of choice, action and engagement across the mouse brain. Nature 576:266–273. https://doi.org/10.1038/s41586-019-1787-x
16. Siegle JH, Jia X, Durand S et al (2021) Survey of spiking in the mouse visual system reveals functional hierarchy. Nature 592:86–92. https://doi.org/10.1038/s41586-020-03171-x
17. Andermann ML, Kerlin AM, Roumis DK et al (2011) Functional specialization of mouse higher visual cortical areas. Neuron 72:1025–1039. https://doi.org/10.1016/j.neuron.2011.11.013
18. Pinto L, Rajan K, DePasquale B et al (2019) Task-dependent changes in the large-scale dynamics and necessity of cortical regions. Neuron 104:810–824.e9. https://doi.org/10.1016/j.neuron.2019.08.025
19. Otazu GH, Chae H, Davis MB, Albeanu DF (2015) Cortical feedback Decorrelates olfactory bulb output in awake mice. Neuron 86: 1461–1477. https://doi.org/10.1016/j.neuron.2015.05.023
20. Bolding KA, Franks KM (2017) Complementary codes for odor identity and intensity in olfactory cortex. eLife 6:e22630. https://doi.org/10.7554/eLife.22630
21. Bolding KA, Franks KM (2018) Recurrent cortical circuits implement concentration-invariant odor coding. Science 361:eaat6904. https://doi.org/10.1126/science.aat6904
22. Bolding KA, Nagappan S, Han B-X et al (2020) Recurrent circuitry is required to stabilize piriform cortex odor representations across brain states. eLife 9:e53125. https://doi.org/10.7554/eLife.53125
23. Pashkovski SL, Iurilli G, Brann D et al (2020) Structure and flexibility in cortical representations of odour space. Nature 583:253–258. https://doi.org/10.1038/s41586-020-2451-1
24. Zak JD, Reddy G, Vergassola M, Murthy VN (2020) Antagonistic odor interactions in olfactory sensory neurons are widespread in freely

breathing mice. Nat Commun 11:3350. https://doi.org/10.1038/s41467-020-17124-5

25. Isaacson JS, Scanziani M (2011) How Inhibition Shapes Cortical Activity Neuron. Cur Biol 72:231–243. https://doi.org/10.1016/j.neuron.2011.09.027
26. Pi H-J, Hangya B, Kvitsiani D et al (2013) Cortical interneurons that specialize in disinhibitory control. Nature 503:521–524. https://doi.org/10.1038/nature12676
27. Kepecs A, Fishell G (2014) Interneuron cell types are fit to function. Nature 505:318–326. https://doi.org/10.1038/nature12983
28. Zeng H, Sanes JR (2017) Neuronal cell-type classification: challenges, opportunities and the path forward. Nat Rev Neurosci 18:530–546. https://doi.org/10.1038/nrn.2017.85
29. Economo MN, Viswanathan S, Tasic B et al (2018) Distinct descending motor cortex pathways and their roles in movement. Nature 563:79–84. https://doi.org/10.1038/s41586-018-0642-9
30. Tasic B, Yao Z, Graybuck LT et al (2018) Shared and distinct transcriptomic cell types across neocortical areas. Nature 563:72–78. https://doi.org/10.1038/s41586-018-0654-5
31. Fox SE, Ranck JB (1975) Localization and anatomical identification of theta and complex spike cells in dorsal hippocampal formation of rats. Exp Neurol 49:299–313. https://doi.org/10.1016/0014-4886(75)90213-7
32. Fox SE, Ranck JB (1981) Electrophysiological characteristics of hippocampal complex-spike cells and theta cells. Exp Brain Res 41:399–410. https://doi.org/10.1007/BF00238898
33. Kubie JL, Muller RU, Bostock E (1990) Spatial firing properties of hippocampal theta cells. J Neurosci 10:1110–1123. https://doi.org/10.1523/JNEUROSCI.10-04-01110.1990
34. Barthó P, Hirase H, Monconduit L et al (2004) Characterization of neocortical principal cells and interneurons by network interactions and extracellular features. J Neurophysiol 92:600–608. https://doi.org/10.1152/jn.01170.2003
35. Fujisawa S, Amarasingham A, Harrison MT, Buzsáki G (2008) Behavior-dependent short-term assembly dynamics in the medial prefrontal cortex. Nat Neurosci 11:823–833. https://doi.org/10.1038/nn.2134
36. English DF, McKenzie S, Evans T et al (2017) Pyramidal cell-interneuron circuit architecture and dynamics in hippocampal networks. Neuron 96:505–520.e7. https://doi.org/10.1016/j.neuron.2017.09.033
37. Lima SQ, Hromádka T, Znamenskiy P, Zador AM (2009) PINP: a new method of tagging neuronal populations for identification during in vivo electrophysiological recording. PLoS One 4:e6099. https://doi.org/10.1371/journal.pone.0006099
38. Cardin JA, Carlén M, Meletis K et al (2010) Targeted optogenetic stimulation and recording of neurons in vivo using cell-type-specific expression of Channelrhodopsin-2. Nat Protoc 5:247–254. https://doi.org/10.1038/nprot.2009.228
39. Zhang S-J, Ye J, Miao C et al (2013) Optogenetic dissection of entorhinal-hippocampal functional connectivity. Science 340:1232627. https://doi.org/10.1126/science.1232627
40. Roux L, Stark E, Sjulson L, Buzsáki G (2014) In vivo optogenetic identification and manipulation of GABAergic interneuron subtypes. Curr Opin Neurobiol 26:88–95. https://doi.org/10.1016/j.conb.2013.12.013
41. Kim CK, Adhikari A, Deisseroth K (2017) Integration of optogenetics with complementary methodologies in systems neuroscience. Nat Rev Neurosci 18:222–235. https://doi.org/10.1038/nrn.2017.15
42. Fenno LE, Mattis J, Ramakrishnan C et al (2014) Targeting cells with single vectors using multiple-feature Boolean logic. Nat Methods 11:763–772. https://doi.org/10.1038/nmeth.2996
43. Fenno LE, Ramakrishnan C, Kim YS et al (2020) Comprehensive dual- and triple-feature intersectional single-vector delivery of diverse functional payloads to cells of behaving mammals. Neuron 107:836–853.e11. https://doi.org/10.1016/j.neuron.2020.06.003
44. Madisen L, Garner AR, Shimaoka D et al (2015) Transgenic mice for intersectional targeting of neural sensors and effectors with high specificity and performance. Neuron 85:942–958. https://doi.org/10.1016/j.neuron.2015.02.022
45. Daigle TL, Madisen L, Hage TA et al (2018) A suite of transgenic driver and reporter mouse lines with enhanced brain-cell-type targeting and functionality. Cell 174:465–480.e22. https://doi.org/10.1016/j.cell.2018.06.035
46. Nagappan S, Franks KM (2021) Parallel processing by distinct classes of principal neurons in the olfactory cortex. eLife 10:e73668. https://doi.org/10.7554/eLife.73668
47. Guo ZV, Hires SA, Li N et al (2014) Procedures for behavioral experiments in head-fixed mice. PLoS One 9:e88678. https://doi.org/10.1371/journal.pone.0088678

48. Barkus C, Bergmann C, Branco T et al (2022) Refinements to rodent head fixation and fluid/food control for neuroscience. J Neurosci Methods 381:109705. https://doi.org/10.1016/j.jneumeth.2022.109705
49. Huber D, Gutnisky DA, Peron S et al (2012) Multiple dynamic representations in the motor cortex during sensorimotor learning. Nature 484:473–478. https://doi.org/10.1038/nature11039
50. Osborne JE, Dudman JT (2014) RIVETS: a mechanical system for in vivo and in vitro electrophysiology and imaging. PLoS One 9:e89007. https://doi.org/10.1371/journal.pone.0089007
51. The International Brain Laboratory, Aguillon-Rodriguez V, Angelaki D et al (2021) Standardized and reproducible measurement of decision-making in mice. eLife 10:e63711. https://doi.org/10.7554/eLife.63711
52. Goldey GJ, Roumis DK, Glickfeld LL et al (2014) Removable cranial windows for long-term imaging in awake mice. Nat Protoc 9:2515–2538. https://doi.org/10.1038/nprot.2014.165
53. Yger P, Spampinato GL, Esposito E et al (2018) A spike sorting toolbox for up to thousands of electrodes validated with ground truth recordings in vitro and in vivo. eLife 7:e34518. https://doi.org/10.7554/eLife.34518
54. Pachitariu M, Sridhar S, Stringer C (2023) Solving the spike sorting problem with Kilosort. bioRxiv, 2023-01. https://doi.org/10.1101/2023.01.07.523036
55. Buccino AP, Hurwitz CL, Garcia S et al (2020) SpikeInterface, a unified framework for spike sorting. eLife 9:e61834. https://doi.org/10.7554/eLife.61834
56. Kvitsiani D, Ranade S, Hangya B et al (2013) Distinct behavioural and network correlates of two interneuron types in prefrontal cortex. Nature 498:363–366. https://doi.org/10.1038/nature12176
57. Wolff SBE, Gründemann J, Tovote P et al (2014) Amygdala interneuron subtypes control fear learning through disinhibition. Nature 509:453–458. https://doi.org/10.1038/nature13258
58. Rowland DC, Obenhaus HA, Skytøen ER et al (2018) Functional properties of stellate cells in medial entorhinal cortex layer II. eLife 7:e36664. https://doi.org/10.7554/eLife.36664

Correction to: Identification and Localization of Cell Types in the Mouse Olfactory Bulb Using Slide-SeqV2

Ai Fang, Kaitlyn Petentler, Andrew Price, Seth Malloy, Michael Peterson, Lucinda Maddera, Jonathon Russell, McKenzie Treese, Hua Li, Yongfu Wang, Sean McKinney, Anoja Perera, and C. Ron Yu

Correction to:
Chapter 13 in: Bradley J. Goldstein, Hiroaki Matsunami (eds.), ***The Olfactory System,*** **Methods in Molecular Biology, vol. 2710,**
https://doi.org/10.1007/978-1-0716-3425-7_13

Chapter 13 was mistakenly published without an author name and with a mistake in another author name. The author names have been updated as below:

Ai Fang, Kaitlyn Petentler, Andrew Price, Seth Malloy, Michael Peterson, Lucinda Maddera, Jonathon Russell, McKenzie Treese, Hua Li, Yongfu Wang, Sean McKinney, Anoja Perera & C. Ron Yu

---

The updated original version of this chapter can be found at
https://doi.org/10.1007/978-1-0716-3425-7_13

Bradley J. Goldstein and Hiroaki Matsunami (eds.), *The Olfactory System*, Methods in Molecular Biology, vol. 2710,
https://doi.org/10.1007/978-1-0716-3425-7_17,

Index

Bradley J. Goldstein and Hiroaki Matsunami (eds.), *The Olfactory System*, Methods in Molecular Biology, vol. 2710, https://doi.org/10.1007/978-1-0716-3425-7,

MIX
Papier aus verantwortungsvollen Quellen
Paper from responsible sources
FSC® C105338
FSC
www.fsc.org

If you have any concerns about our products,
you can contact us on
ProductSafety@springernature.com

In case Publisher is established outside the EU,
the EU authorized representative is:
Springer Nature Customer Service Center GmbH
Europaplatz 3, 69115 Heidelberg, Germany

Printed by Libri Plureos GmbH
in Hamburg, Germany